WORKING WITH ELDERLY PEOPLE

HUMAN HORIZONS SERIES

WORKING WITH ELDERLY PEOPLE

A. MURPHY

A CONDOR BOOK
SOUVENIR PRESS (E&A) LTD

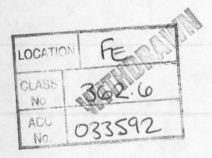

CONTENTS

ACKNOWLEDGEMENTS

I should like to thank the following people who have helped to make this book possible:

Jean Allen, Incontinence Advisor, Community Unit, Sheffield Health Authority;

Barbara Dixon, Senior Occupational Therapist (Elderly Mentally Infirm), Northern General Hospital, Sheffield;

Elizabeth Highfield, Chief Audiology Technician, Royal Hallamshire Hospital, Sheffield;

Janet Hogger, Community Physiotherapist, Community Unit, Sheffield Health Authority;

Isobel O'Leary, Senior Speech and Language Therapist, Royal Hallamshire Hospital, Sheffield;

Kevin Price, Mobility Officer for the Blind, Sheffield Family and Community Services Department;

and also other staff who have read this book.

I am also grateful to the following for permission to use copyright illustrations:

Handicapped Living Centre, Sheffield, for drawings of walking aids and a table; Academic Press for drawings of a walking frame in use from *An Outline of Geriatrics* by H.M. Hodgkinson; Churchill Livingstone for drawings of going up and down stairs and fitting and propelling a wheelchair from *The Practice of Occupational Therapy* by Ann Turner; Everest & Jennings Inc. for drawings showing how to negotiate stairs with a wheelchair from their booklet *Wheelchair Owner's Manual*; The Disability Information Trust for 14 drawings on using a wheelchair from *Wheelchairs* (5th edition); The Department of Health for a drawing of a wheelchair footplate from *Hints on the Use of Your Wheelchair*; J. & P. Coats for drawings of crochet and embroidery stitches from their booklets; Boxtree for three drawings of a bottle garden from *Gardening Time* by William Davidson (Tiger Books); Horticultural Therapy for five drawings from *Able to Garden* by P. Please (Batsford); Age Concern for three drawings from *Gardening in Retirement* by Isobel Pays.

Finally I should like to thank RADAR for allowing me to use the chart reproduced on p. 46 from their book *Choosing a Wheelchair*.

A.M.

PREFACE

Staff working in day centres, residential homes and other units for elderly people have often expressed a need for a book that brings together helpful information and ideas. This collection of notes was compiled while working in a day centre with elderly people who had a range of different physical conditions. It was originally prepared for new staff who were starting work in a centre for the first time and was intended as a simple introduction to some of the activities that could be used there.

At the same time it seemed a good idea to provide some information about the running of a centre and about the elderly people who use it. When working with people who may be frail both physically and mentally staff need to know how to handle and communicate with them, how to help them cope with their disabilities and what to do in an emergency. Some basic information about the disorders of old age is essential. This is discussed in the first part of the book.

The second part covers the activities. These are not intended as 'treatment' but to provide interests, entertainment and mental stimulation. They can all be done easily in a centre, and many are pastimes and hobbies that elderly people may choose to do for themselves.

In the Appendices are suggestions for further sources of information, including books, addresses of suppliers and societies and sources of help.

I hope that you will find the notes helpful and of benefit. If you would like to make any comments, these would be welcomed.

A.M.

The writers regret that they cannot
accept responsibility for any
incidents, accidents, injuries or
other damages to persons or property
arising from the use of information,
procedures, aids or equipment
mentioned in this book.

Part One

BASIC INFORMATION

1 CENTRES, STAFF AND CLIENTS

In this book the word 'centre' has been used to mean anywhere where elderly people may meet together—a group run by volunteers, a luncheon club, a day centre, a residential home, nursing home or other long-stay unit.

A day centre is a place where they can go for a few hours during the day to enjoy social or recreational activities, whether for one day a week or more often, either on a weekday or at the weekend. The centre may be used by people who have a mental or physical disability or special needs, or simply by those who would benefit from company, a meal, bathing, hairdressing, counselling, advice or any other support. Carers may also appreciate having respite from an elderly relative. Other services which may be available could include nursing, chiropody, social work, physiotherapy, occupational therapy and so on.

Day centres may be managed by a Local Authority, voluntary organisation or by a private concern, or they may be run by volunteers from a local charity, church or community group. They may be held in a community centre or church hall, in adapted premises or in a specially built centre, or they may be part of a residential home or other unit.

The type of staff in the centre will depend on the organisation that is responsible for running it. If it is managed by a Local Authority or an institution there could be paid staff who have had training and experience in providing the different services; if it is run by a local voluntary group the services offered may be more limited.

The atmosphere should be as happy and relaxed as possible, so that the elderly people can feel free to enjoy themselves and take part in any of the activities which may be available. These should be suited to the abilities of those who attend and should also be of benefit to them, providing interest and stimulation.

In some centres the elderly people who go there may not be mobile or may live some distance away, so that transport will have to be arranged. This may be by ambulance or an adapted vehicle (one which will take wheelchairs), or taxis and cars can be used if people can manage these easily. In some areas special transport schemes for elderly and disabled people may be available, or 'friends' of the centre may have contributed towards a minibus which may be shared with other centres.

From time to time it will be necessary to check how the centre is running and whether it is keeping up with its aims, and to ensure that the people who attend are benefiting from being there.

THE LAYOUT OF A CENTRE

If a centre is to be used by people with a physical disability, it may need to be adapted so that it will be safe and suitable for them. This could mean providing level access from the road, doorways and fire exits that are wide enough to take the widest wheelchair (with a person propelling it himself), handrails in convenient places such as on door jambs, along corridors, beside steps and in toilet and bathing areas, and also enough space for someone to turn and use a wheelchair in a confined space like a toilet. If there are people with a visual impairment who walk unaided, it may be necessary to provide continuous handrails around the centre.

Furniture and fittings also need to be appropriate for the people who attend, and in a centre for elderly people these could include a selection of armchairs at different heights. Vinyl coverings on chairs help to protect them from damage or stains, and sometimes additional cushions or supports can be added to make the sitter more comfortable or secure. If stacking chairs are used these may also need to have armrests. Footstools are used in some centres.

Tables should be suitable for the particular activities—for example, occasional tables can be used for reading magazines, while work tables should be at a convenient height for the people using them, whether they are standing or sitting down in a chair or wheelchair. Sometimes tables have to be stackable if space is limited.

Floors must be safe to walk on, and non-slip floor coverings or fitted short-pile carpets will help to prevent people from falling, although coverings on which the feet tend to 'stick' may be hazardous. If drinks, food or urine are likely to be spilt on the floor, Flotex carpets or surfaces that are easy to clean will have to be used.

If a centre is on more than one level it may be necessary to install a ramp (minimum 1 in 12) or a lift or stairlift to provide access to another storey, but ordinary stairs may be adequate if the elderly people are agile enough to use them.

In areas where people may fall easily, such as toilets, alarms may be needed, and also outward-opening doors and locks that can be operated from the outside. Additional aids such as raised toilet seats and free-standing toilet frames can be added later, and hoists and commode chairs which fit over toilets can be made available if these are needed.

Wheelchairs, walking aids and other equipment can be kept in a storage area when not in use; this may need to be locked at night if the centre is also used by other groups for different purposes.

Other facilities which may be needed include a dining-room, a lounge/TV room, a games room, quiet/rest room, chiropody and treatment room, bathroom, hairdressing area and places for other activities. The outside of the building must allow easy access for people who are both elderly and disabled from either ambulances or public transport, and seats should be provided inside and outside for those who are only able to walk short distances.

If a building has very narrow corridors that do not allow wheelchairs to be manoeuvred, or would require major adaptations such as the installation of a lift, it would be worthwhile looking for different accommodation which would be easier to use.

PROVIDING CARE

As we have seen, a centre designed for elderly people must be safe, easy to use and accessible. Good lighting is also essential, as well as adequate ventilation and enough heating to ensure that the room temperature is comfortable for people who are likely to be sitting down for most of the day.

The elderly people may need to be encouraged to use the furniture and equipment that is most suited to their particular needs—for example, a chair of the right height and size, or a table which is at a convenient working height for any given activity. If a person needs a cushion, staff will need to find out which is the most appropriate one to use. The local occupational therapist, Disabled Living Centre or District Health Authority

14

should be able to advise about this, and it may be worthwhile having a selection of different cushions in the centre, so that clients can try them out and choose the one they prefer. Some people may also want a rug, footstool, incontinence cover and so on.

Many elderly people are able to look after themselves without any assistance, while others may depend on staff for quite a lot of their needs. Despite this, they should be encouraged to be as independent as possible while engaged in activities that they can do safely.

In any centre, it is helpful if members of staff can work together as a team. This not only improves their efficiency but also benefits the service being provided and helps staff to feel that they are making a real contribution to the running of the centre. Staff meetings can also be used as a means of raising issues and discussing problems and progress.

Any centre must follow the Health and Safety regulations so that staff, elderly people and any visitors are not at risk. These will probably have been drawn up by the organisation responsible for the running of the centre and should be kept in a place where all staff can read them. In a centre run by volunteers there may be no existing regulations, and a set of appropriate guidelines will need to be obtained (the local Social Services Department may be able to help).

VOLUNTARY WORKERS

Volunteers can contribute a great deal to a centre—by assisting the staff and elderly people, or by doing tasks around the unit. This will improve the service and also enable the staff to provide additional activities.

Staff need to be careful when accepting volunteers and should check that they are suitable for work in a centre with elderly people. This may mean using the same procedures as with the paid staff—filling in an application form (with the names of two people willing to give a reference) and attending for an interview. This is important, particularly if the volunteer is going to drive, handle money or be alone with the elderly people.

The application form can be quite simple (see p. 17) and the interview informal, but staff need to know whether the person is in good health mentally and physically, and whether she will be able to undertake whatever work she may be asked to do. She should also be genuinely interested in elderly people and be able to communicate and work with them. During the interview she may ask to look round the centre, meet the elderly people and see what kind of activities she will be doing. She may enquire about supervision and training, and also about the reimbursement of expenses.

When taking on volunteers it is important to review the Health and Safety provisions and to find out whether the volunteer and centre are covered by insurance. This may be needed if the volunteer is involved in an accident and should cover all contingencies—her own fault or someone else's, injury to herself, an elderly person, a member of staff or the general public, and loss or damage to property. Accidents can happen in many different ways. A minibus or piece of equipment may be poorly maintained or faulty; the volunteer may have had insufficient supervision or training, or an elderly person may be awkward to manage. Volunteer drivers should find out whether their motor insurance covers the work for the centre—some insurance companies will provide this cover at no extra cost.

To avoid an accident happening, staff must follow the Health and Safety policy of the centre and be aware of any guidelines when dealing with volunteers. These should include ensuring that they are capable of doing all the activities required of them, providing adequate supervision and training and checking that the volunteer knows where her responsibility ends. The volunteer should know who is supervising her, and whom to contact for support, information and training. This may be a Voluntary Services Organiser or a member of staff in the centre.

A fund should be maintained to pay the expenses of any volunteers who may be out of pocket through visiting the centre.

ELDERLY PEOPLE

A person is usually regarded as 'elderly' when he or she has reached retirement age, although how someone performs mentally or physically will vary from one individual to another—some are quite young at 70 while others are 'old' at a much younger age. This may cause problems in a day centre when staff have to try and decide who should attend: some centres will only accept people up to the age of 60 or 65, while others will not take people under retirement age.

As people grow older they may no longer be able to take part in activities which they could do previously; this may be due to failing eyesight, reduced hearing, forgetfulness, limited concentration, anxiety, confusion, loss of confidence or interest, or because they have a particular complaint that affects their ability to perform a task, such as pain, stiffness, deformity, immobility, weakness, discomfort, breathlessness, depression and so on (see Appendices for list of conditions).

Older people may also be affected by events and circumstances such as bereavement, isolation, poor home conditions, restricted environment, altered home circumstances, poverty, poor diet, loss of independence, constant admissions to hospital, lack of support from family and friends, and perhaps also lack of support and advice from Health and Social Services.

How a person copes with the different situations may depend upon his or her previous attitudes and expectations—some people may be able to accept change while others may become aggressive, agitated, unco-operative, withdrawn or depressed.

Sometimes an elderly person has to decide whether to move into a long-stay unit and this can be a difficult time, often associated with the death of a partner, sudden disability, deteriorating mental or physical condition, or simply because a carer or support services are no longer able to cope with the situation. When the decision has been made, the elderly person has to adjust to the loss of his or her own home and become familiar with new surroundings, people and routines. It may mean having to adapt to some loss of privacy and learning to live with other people.

Staff need to be aware of any difficulties that the elderly person may be experiencing, so that they can give support and encouragement and provide help in overcoming them.

INTERVIEWING CLIENTS

How an elderly person is approached on his or her first day can be very important. Those who have never heard of or attended a centre before may feel quite shy and nervous and could easily be upset by being addressed rather sharply or abruptly. Initially, nothing more than a general introduction will be needed, but later it may be necessary to ask a few simple questions, particularly if very little is known about the person—name, address, date of birth, condition, any medication and details about the client's doctor, social worker and next of kin. If the next of kin is a relative living some distance away, it may be useful to have a note about friends and neighbours living locally, and their whereabouts during the day and at night.

VOLUNTARY SERVICES

Dear . . . .   Date . . . .

Thank you for offering to visit our centre as a volunteer. We need to provide information about our volunteers and it would be appreciated if you could let us have the following details about yourself:

Name: Address: Telephone No.:   Date of birth:
Have you any experience with the elderly or special skills or interests?
Can you give the names of two people who would be willing to give you a reference?
Would you like to help with any of these activities? (please tick)   ☐ reading to the elderly   ☐ driving the minibus   ☐ talking to the elderly   ☐ helping with outings   ☐ helping the staff   ☐ film or slide shows   ☐ refreshments   ☐ concerts   ☐ fund-raising   ☐ sing-songs   ☐ helping with events   ☐ playing the piano   ☐ games   ☐ music   ☐ craftwork   ☐ socials or parties   ☐ gardening   ☐ outdoor activities   ☐ other activities:
Are there any particular days or times which are most convenient for you?

I hope that you will enjoy coming to our centre,

Yours sincerely,
Manager, Broadlands Centre

Please return to the Voluntary Services Organiser, Social Services Dept

If the elderly person seems a little overwhelmed, it may be a good idea to suggest that you would like to ask him some simple questions later on, so that he is prepared. Sometimes you may be asked why the questions have to be answered, and it will help to have some short answer ready.

Information from interviews will need to be written down later in a client's file or notes and any other details added when necessary. It is important for essential notes to be quickly and easily read! Try to avoid writing too much in front of the person you are questioning, although you may have to jot down a few brief notes.

When asking about a person and his condition, you should find out all that will affect your care and treatment of him while he is attending the centre, but irrelevant questions should be avoided. In some centres, staff may be able to get information from a doctor, social worker or another member of staff, but in other instances it may be necessary to question the person himself. Staff need to be aware that an elderly person's account of his own condition and medication is not always accurate or reliable and that they may still have to contact a doctor if they have any queries. Details about medication are important, particularly if a person has to take this during his stay in the centre. Elderly people with conditions such as diabetes, epilepsy or heart and chest complaints may need special attention from the staff. Other information you may need could include special diets, need for regular toileting and any special procedures, arrangements or aids which the person may need to use.

Interests, hobbies and past occupations are a useful guide for any member of staff who is responsible for organising activities and encouraging the elderly people to take part in them.

If the centre is not a residential one, staff will also need to make arrangements for transporting the person to and from the centre and also for contacting any relations or neighbours if a person is unable to attend. These points should be raised during your chat.

When interviewing an elderly person it is important to pick a suitable time and place so that he or she feels relaxed and is able to talk freely. Any personal information disclosed during the interview should be confidential to the staff who need to know it and should be kept in a place where it cannot be seen by others attending the centre.

A sample of a typical referral or interview form is given opposite.

SOCIAL SERVICES DEPARTMENT
DAY CENTRES

Centre: Date:

Name:

Address: Date of birth:

Case Number:

Marital State:

Next of Kin, or person to be   Social Worker/
contacted in an emergency: Welfare Asst:

Name: Area:

Address: G.P.:
Address:

Tel. no: Tel. No:

Disability:

Any special medication or precautions:

Past Employment:

Interests/Hobbies:

Notes:

This client is to attend the centre on   days and
will travel by   transport.
He/she started at the centre on   and is non/ambulant.
Notes overleaf.

2 IMPAIRING CONDITIONS

STROKE

A stroke is caused by an interruption of the blood supply to the brain. This may be due to a haemorrhage or a blood clot, or it may be the result of an injury. It can affect either side of the body and there may be different symptoms such as partial or complete paralysis (hemiplegia), difficulty in maintaining posture, balance or walking, incontinence, drooping mouth, dribbling, difficulty in swallowing, inability to speak normally and perhaps problems in understanding speech as well. 'Unseen' symptoms may include a change in personality, confusion, disorientation, limited concentration, poor memory, inattention, lack of awareness of the body or disability, visual problems, impaired sensation, emotional instability and so on.

Some people may be able to accept what has happened and try to lead a normal life again (if this is possible), but others may have difficulty in adjusting to the situation and become dependent, anxious, depressed, unco-operative, resentful or aggressive.

If a person's arm or hand has become affected by a stroke, it may be possible to position it for him if he is unable to do this for himself—for example, it may be 'tight', with the shoulder drooping and the elbow, wrist and fingers flexed, or it may hang loosely down by his side. Sometimes one hand or arm may tighten up if he is doing something with the other which he finds demanding or difficult or if he is under stress, and staff will need to try to persuade him to rest or to do an activity that is easier, or to find out why he is distressed.

When someone with a stroke has to be lifted, staff may decide to do a 'stroke lift' if this is suitable and the person is not too heavy or awkward. If two members of staff are lifting him, the one on the affected side should support the shoulder with care so that it does not become damaged by the lift (see *The Handling of Patients: A guide for nurses* in FURTHER READING).

If he wants to use a chair, it is important to check that it is stable, comfortable and supporting and has a seat that will allow him to sit well back while keeping his feet flat on the floor. He will have to try to keep a normal sitting position with his weight taken evenly on both hips. If he is using a wheelchair, the footplates may need adjusting so that he can keep his knees and ankles at right angles, and any movable parts, such as armrests, legrests and so on, must be in place. A cushion may be used if he is uncomfortable, likely to develop pressure areas or if he needs to be higher in the chair.

If a table is being used, this may have to be adjusted to the right height so that he can rest his forearms on it comfortably and keep a good sitting position.

In some centres there may be a physiotherapist available to help with positioning and walking, and an occupational therapist who can advise about aids and equipment. If the elderly person has difficulty in communicating or is in need of an aid, a speech therapist will be able to provide help.

Sitting in a chair

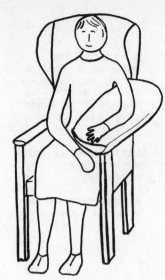

Chair giving support.

Pillow supporting the affected arm.

Person comfortable in the chair.

Chair the right height with the feet flat on the floor.

Chair not giving enough support.

Arm has become bent and 'tight'.

Person tending to fall sideways.

Foot not flat on the floor.

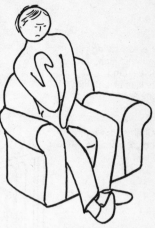

Being pushed in a wheelchair

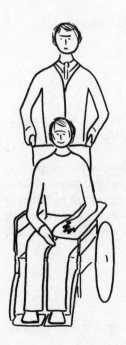

Person sitting upright in the wheelchair with the affected arm being supported on a Bexhill armrest.

Person is comfortable and the footrests have been adjusted to the right height.

(Note: A person needs to be assessed by an occupational therapist or physiotherapist before using a Bexhill armrest.)

Attendant unaware of what is happening.

Affected hand becoming trapped in the wheel.

Armrest missing —person could fall out sideways and his cover could get caught in the wheel.

Footrest is missing and the affected leg is being dragged under the wheelchair.

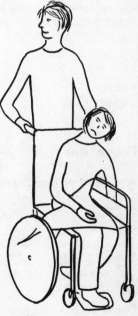

A person who has had a stroke sitting at a table

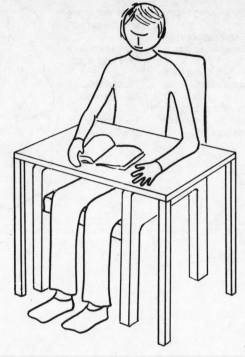

Person sitting with his hips, knees and ankles at a right angle.

Chair at the right height from the floor.

Arm and hand held comfortably on a table of the right height (a piece of non-slip material may be needed under the arm to prevent it from slipping off the table).

Hand held flat on the table with the fingers outstretched.

An adjustable table may be useful in some centres.

Feet flat on the floor.

Table needs to be deep enough so that the elbow or hand do not fall off it.

NOTE: Do not try to move the arm if it is liable to be uncomfortable, painful or 'too tight'. If this is likely to happen, leave it on a pillow—ask advice from a physiotherapist if one is available.

Aids

Identity card —An identity card can be used if a person is unable to give his name and address. It is available from the Stroke Association.

Picture book —Pictures or drawings of activities or things which a person may need can be put together in a small photograph album.

Word and picture chart—This chart is useful if someone is able to point out pictures or spell words. It has a clock, alphabet, days and months and also pictures of everyday activities. It is available from the Stroke Association.

DEMENTIA
by Barbara Dixon

Dementia is a progressive condition in which brain cells die more rapidly than normal. This causes a gradual decline in the sufferer's abilities. There is no cure.

Most people who are affected are elderly. It is not an inevitable part of growing old, but may be caused by several disease processes. By far the most common are Alzheimer's Disease, in which the memory, personality and intellectual abilities are affected, and 'multi-infarct dementia' which is caused by a number of small strokes blocking the blood supply to areas of the brain. The cause of Alzheimer's Disease is unknown.

Any person who appears to be confused must be referred to a doctor. There are other medical and psychiatric disorders which can present symptoms very similar to those of dementing illnesses, so it is important that the person has a diagnosis and is given appropriate treatment. Although dementing illnesses are not curable, the doctor may be able to recommend treatment which might relieve some of the symptoms. When a person becomes confused very suddenly, the symptoms may be due to a toxic confusional state caused by a physical illness. If this is the case, the symptoms can disappear after a doctor has prescribed appropriate treatment.

Typically, the onset of dementia is gradual. At first the sufferer may appear less able to concentrate, make choices and adapt to change, becoming forgetful and less able to cope with the routine activities of daily living. Often he realises that his abilities are declining and may find this very distressing. As time passes his forgetfulness increases, he puts himself in unsafe situations and becomes muddled about time and place. He may develop communication problems, restlessness and behave inappropriately, becoming easily upset and sometimes aggressive. Some people also suffer from hallucinations. Eventually a person may be unable to recognise even close relatives or to make sense of the world around him, and he may become completely dependent on others.

The notes that follow discuss ways of approaching some of the common problems that may be caused by the symptoms of dementia.

Memory problems

The short-term memory is affected first. The person loses the ability to remember what has just happened to him, which can cause a lot of practical problems. He may be unable to remember whether he has just eaten and either go out without food or prepare meals far more often than he needs. He may forget to wash and change his clothes regularly, or keep repeating the same simple task such as dusting, whilst forgetting to do other equally important jobs. Often he may hide items safely, but forget where. This sometimes leads to accusations of stealing. Repetition of the same statements and questions is common and can be extremely wearing to carers. Poor memory causes learning difficulties—the person loses the ability to learn behaviour which might otherwise relieve his problems and improve independence.

Sometimes memory aids such as lists, clocks, calendars and notices are useful. These should be as large and simple as possible to enable people to use them effectively. Staff should point out cues frequently to help forgetful people become accustomed to using them. They should try to explain what is happening patiently and reassuringly to people who are repetitive, and consider whether there are ways of distracting them from such behaviour.

Long-term memory is retained longer than short-term memory. A person may be able to remember a lot of information from the past and hold long and interesting conversations about it, but be unable to tell you what happened minutes ago. Different skills are involved. A good long-term memory does not indicate that a person is pretending if her conversation is repetitive or if she cannot tell you what she had for lunch.

Orientation problems

People with dementing illnesses become disorientated in time, so that they are unable to decide what time of day it is, or what week or year. This often causes inappropriate behaviour—for example, constantly asking the time or sleeping through the day, but remaining awake and active at night. Many have difficulty in remembering where they are and where their home is, or become incapable of finding their way around, even in very familiar places. Most people experience difficulty in putting names to new faces and recognising friends whom they do not see often; some eventually lose the ability to recognise people who have been close to them for many years. This can be very distressing, both for the sufferer and for the family.

Communication problems

Many people with dementia develop language problems and may lose the ability to express themselves lucidly. Some sufferers will be aware of this and become frustrated because they cannot make their needs understood; others may not realise that their attempts at speech do not make sense to the hearer, and will wonder why carers are unable to respond appropriately to their needs. Many lose the ability to understand language and so can no longer follow instructions.

Continue to speak to a person who develops language problems. Explain exactly what is happening. Use short, simple phrases and rephrase them if the person does not understand. Speak simply and clearly. Avoid shouting or speaking exaggeratedly slowly, as this disturbs the natural rhythm of speech, making it harder to understand. Do not assume that a person who is unable to express himself clearly cannot understand you either. Always try to communicate with people who do not appear to understand, as they may take in a little of what you are saying and most will appreciate the effort you are making to communicate effectively. Use gesture and facial expressions to clarify your message. Short, well-written messages may occasionally be helpful, too. Poor hearing is likely to be the problem, rather than language difficulties, if writing seems to be particularly helpful.

A lot of communication abilities in elderly people are inhibited simply because they are not using hearing aids, spectacles, false teeth or mobility aids which would help them to gain more information from their environment, move about more easily and articulate more effectively. This applies as much to people with dementia as to anyone else. So if a person appears to need aids, get these assessed and fitted properly and encourage him always to use any aid that is recommended. Sometimes a person with dementia will be unable to adapt and learn to use an otherwise suitable aid effectively.

Deterioration in intellectual abilities

This leads to errors of judgement, and to difficulty in deciding what is significant and in making choices, which can lead to a lot of problems. For instance, crossing the road or cooking a meal can become hazardous and may lead to loss of independence.

Try to keep the environment simple and restrict decisions to those with which the patient can cope, whilst encouraging him to exercise some choice—for example, limit his choice of coats, or items on a menu, to two or three, so that he is not overwhelmed by a wide range of options.

Review the safety policy regularly to ensure that the unit is as safe as it can be whilst still allowing all users the opportunity to exercise as much freedom as possible. There is always some risk in allowing people to make their own choices—and their own errors. The balance between providing a safe environment and one that allows personal freedom can be delicate.

Wandering and restlessness

Many people who suffer from dementia tend to wander around their home or day centre. Some may regularly try to leave, but are unsure where they are going or how to get there.

It is important to establish why such behaviour occurs. If a person wants to go out, is still able to find his way back, is mobile and retains a good road sense, he is not 'wandering' at all and should be able to come and go as he pleases. If his wish to leave is based on muddled ideas and misconceptions, or he is disorientated, try to explain to him where he is and what is happening, or try to distract him.

There are various door catches available, which make it harder for people to leave premises without being noticed. These may interfere with the independence of more able people, so the needs of all centre users must be considered.

If a person constantly wanders inside his home or the centre and this is fatiguing or distressing for him or disturbs others, try to find ways to distract him or work off surplus energy through simple activities or by spending more time with staff. Supervised walks, or opportunities to take part in supervised exercises and active games and dancing will provide an interest for many, and the chance to use excess energy in socially acceptable situations.

Incontinence of urine and faeces

There are many reasons why a person becomes incontinent (see INCONTINENCE, p. 27). Establish the cause so that you can work out how best to manage the problem. A lot of medical causes are treatable. Many confused people become incontinent because they cannot find their way to the toilet or cannot adjust their own clothing. Some people urinate in inappropriate places because they no longer recognise a toilet—for example, they may use a wash basin or a waste bin. Those who have mobility problems may not be able to reach a toilet quickly enough, while others lose the ability to recognise the physical signs that tell them they need to use a toilet.

A lot of incontinence problems can be avoided or improved by regularly reminding, directing or taking a person to the toilet and finding a routine that suits the individual. Incontinence aids such as plastic pants and pads are not always helpful for confused people who may not be able to accept that they are incontinent, or to understand why they are wearing such garments.

Undressing

This can be very embarrassing and difficult for others to understand. Try to communicate to the sufferer that undressing is inappropriate in company. Remind him where he is and what is happening. Undressing may be a sign with some people that they need to be taken to the toilet—or have already been incontinent and are now uncomfortable. Occasionally a person may simply dislike the clothes he is wearing, may not recognise garments as his own, or may feel uncomfortable in a particular outfit.

Aggression and resistiveness

Aggression may be verbal or physical. Often people are aggressive only when they are being given basic care. A dementing person may not recognise this as care at all, but see it as unnecessary interference or even as an assault which he is resisting. A great deal of aggressive behaviour is due to misinterpretation of events.

Again it is important to observe which circumstances cause the behaviour so that all possible steps can be taken to eliminate 'trigger' situations. Try to be calm and matter-of-fact; avoid making the situation worse. Challenging or remonstrating with a violent

25

person may intensify the behaviour. Try to direct the aggressive person away from the situation and explain what is happening if he is willing to listen. Distract him and try to focus his attention on a different activity. There is rarely any point in trying to discuss the incident with a forgetful person later on. Memory problems may prove to be useful here, as he may forget his anger very quickly. Other people who may not have been involved may need a lot of reassurance about aggressive incidents.

When managing people with dementia and encouraging them to maintain their independence, it is important to try to understand the nature of dementia and view each individual as a whole and unique person. Often they are unable to express all their needs and anxieties, and it is important, when their behaviour causes problems to themselves and others, to observe them closely in order to find out what causes difficult behaviour. Staff can then try to work out a consistent approach which they can all use to avoid such behaviour. Ensure that any physical ailments or sudden changes of behaviour are reported to the person's doctor so that any treatment can be considered promptly. Even very minor ailments can greatly increase the levels of confusion and distress in an individual. Also try to encourage each person's positive contributions, however limited, to the life of the unit.

Many centres and residential homes are not specifically designed for elderly people who are mentally ill, and have low staff/resident ratios. It is vital that all staff act consistently towards any confused person to help him understand what everyone expects of him and to help him feel secure. Staff should also remember that new arrivals may take several weeks to settle down and adjust to finding themselves in a new environment; initially troublesome behaviour is to be expected.

Structured activities with elderly mentally ill people

Many forgetful people respond well to a highly structured environment and to taking part in well supervised activities. These need to be kept simple. Except in the very early stages, people are unlikely to have the motivation to organise their own interests.

Exercises, going out for walks, dancing, and indoor games such as 'target games' and skittles, are enjoyed by a surprisingly large number of elderly people and most games can be organised so that participants join in from seated positions if necessary. For people with communication problems, such games provide a social situation in which they can take part easily and can communicate effectively using non-verbal skills. They also provide an acceptable channel for excess energy and help to maintain general fitness. They *must* be well supervised.

Possibly some people could be involved in simple tasks necessary to the running of the unit, such as washing up, cleaning ornaments, laying tables, baking cakes or biscuits for tea, being present and involved when their rooms are tidied and making their own beds. It must be accepted that this is likely to slow down the rate at which staff can work and that tasks will need supervision and checking to ensure that hygiene and safety are maintained.

Most craft activities are really quite complicated procedures, so be careful to choose those that can be broken down into a few simple stages, such as making posters or decorations for their own or shared rooms.

Table games such as dominoes and cards are often very familiar, and large, brightly coloured sets of the most popular games can be obtained easily. A lot of people respond well to music and, even if they have communication difficulties, find that they can remember the words of popular songs. Manicure and hairdressing provide an opportunity for close individual contact with staff. Those who still converse well may also enjoy discussions and quizzes. These can be very hard work for the staff. It is useful to have a stock of ideas, pictures, books and objects which can help to focus attention and stimulate conversation. Many people particularly enjoy reminiscing about the past (see RECALL, p. 127).

In most activities, the number of participants should be kept very small, since disorientated people easily lose concentration, get distracted or wander away if they do not get a high input of staff attention. Most activities are more enjoyable and easier to organise if carried out in a separate, quiet and comfortable room—this minimises distractions and interruptions. At least two members of staff should be present to run a group effectively so that they can support each other in this difficult but rewarding task, deal with distractions and attend to individual needs without disrupting the main activity. Groups like these need to be planned carefully and carried out regularly if they are to be really enjoyable and effective.

INCONTINENCE

In a centre for elderly people, some may have a problem with incontinence, when control of the bladder or bowels (or both) is weakened or lost. It may be caused by a temporary illness, conditions affecting the bladder, infection, disease or injury to the spinal cord, constipation, infection in the urine or following a stroke and in other conditions. In many elderly people it may be the result of immobility, difficulty in using the toilet or in adjusting clothing. Sometimes psychological problems, such as depression, anxiety or bereavement, can cause incontinence.

Types of incontinence

Stress incontinence is brought on by physical or sudden exertion, such as jumping, coughing, sneezing or laughing, and tends to be more common in women.

Urge incontinence happens when an elderly person has an urgent warning that he needs to pass urine, but does not have enough time to reach the toilet. This may occur in a man who has an enlarged prostate gland.

Overflow incontinence occurs when only part of the urine is passed while the person is using the toilet. This is caused by a bladder muscle which is not functioning properly or by a weak sphincter muscle at the bladder outlet, or both. It can be associated with diabetes or constipation, and also with certain diseases that affect the brain or spinal cord, such as a stroke or multiple sclerosis.

Reflex incontinence is a sudden flow of urine without warning.

If a person has an incontinence problem and has not had any medical advice, it is advisable that he should see a doctor who may refer him to a clinic or an incontinence adviser who specialises in the needs of people who have an incontinence problem. Various aids are available, and many elderly people do need guidance on the most suitable aid or appliance for their needs. Some of the aids include:

    commodes
    bedpans
    urinals (male or female)
    non-spill valves (for male urinals)
    catheters
    body-worn appliances
    bidet 'shells' which fit into normal toilets
    pants which hold removable plastic-backed pads

water-repellant duvets

pillow covers

absorbant washable bed and seat pads (which can also be worn on a car seat)

plastic covers for mattresses

Often, when a person is incontinent, different procedures can be used to encourage him to be more continent—for example, appropriate toileting times; controlling the intake of fluids which affect bladder function, such as large amounts of strong coffee, tea, orange juice, Coca-Cola or alcohol; encouraging pelvic floor exercises; making the toilet or commode more accessible; fitting alarm systems or aids; altering clothing so that it is easier to use. If a person is wearing a catheter and drainage bag, the bag will need to be emptied at regular intervals by releasing the valve at the bottom of the bag. Holsters or supports are available to hold a catheter bag.

If the centre is likely to be used by people who may have a problem with incontinence, it is advisable to have vinyl-covered chairs which can be washed down easily. If other chairs are already in use, a Unipad seat pad can be used, although this will need to be washed and dried regularly.

3 MOBILITY

Some elderly people have difficulty in moving about safely, and in order to overcome this they may have been issued with a walking aid. This can help to reduce pain, improve mobility, increase confidence and prevent them from falling.

Walking aids are available from several sources. They may be provided by a hospital department, a hospital or community physiotherapist or a Social Services department, or they can be purchased from shops selling aids. Some authorities loan out aids for a certain time and ask for them to be renewed periodically, or returned if no longer needed.

There is a wide variety of walking aids, including walking sticks, tripod sticks (with three feet), tetrapod sticks (with four feet), crutches for use under the arm or to support the forearm (elbow crutches) and walking frames with or without wheels. Some walking frames can be folded so that they will fit into the boot of a car, or have a seat and a bag or basket to carry objects. Aids can be either fixed or adjustable in height.

Because of the wide range available, it is important for an elderly person to have the right one to suit his particular needs. In a hospital or community setting this assessment is likely to be carried out by a physiotherapist who will also give advice on using the aid. If it has been bought privately, borrowed or obtained by some other means, the aid may not be appropriate to the needs of the person and he may not be using it correctly. For example, if it is too high he will be unable to use it effectively, and if it is too low he will be encouraged to stoop. If staff suspect this, or if a person's condition has deteriorated to such an extent that his aid is no longer suitable, it may be possible to ask for an assessment.

In a centre or home the elderly person will need to be able to use his walking aid easily and safely. The floor should be level and not slippery; carpets must be fixed and, if fitted, should be level with any thresholds under doors. Furniture or other obstacles may have to be moved to allow for the normal use of a walking frame or other aids.

Rubber ferrules are usually fitted onto the ends of walking aids to prevent them from slipping. These are available in different sizes and a ferrule of the appropriate size should be fitted securely onto each end to replace the original ferrules when they begin to wear.

As walking aids are provided to suit the needs of the individual, it is advisable for everyone to use his or her own aid and to keep it nearby, ready for when it is required. Name tags or other markings will help in identification.

All equipment must be checked regularly to ensure that it is in good working order, and if staff find that an aid is damaged or worn, it should be repaired by someone trained to do this, or replaced if necessary.

If staff have a problem with a mobility aid it may be possible to contact a local Disabled Living Centre or physiotherapist for advice.

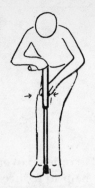

Adjusting an adjustable walking stick
Hold the handle of the stick in one hand and support the lower end if possible. Press in the two spring buttons with the other hand and raise or lower the top end of the stick until the handle is level with the crease in the wrist of the user when he is in a standing position. Allow both buttons to come out fully through the new holes before use.

WALKING AIDS

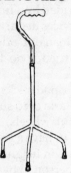

Tripod stick.

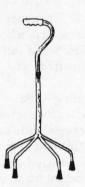

Quadruped or tetrapod stick.

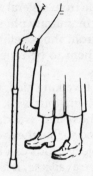

Adjustable walking stick.

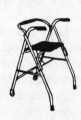

'A' walking frame with seat—this can be folded.

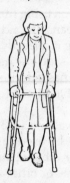

Adjustable walking frame.

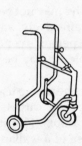

Delta walking aid with wheels.

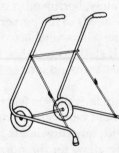

Rollator walking frame (this model can be folded).

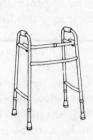

Folding adjustable walking frame.

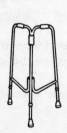

Alpha adjustable walking frame—this can be folded.

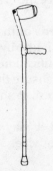

Adjustable elbow crutch.

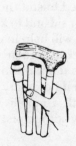

Folding walking stick.

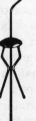

Rest stick and walking stick (the seat folds back when used as a walking stick).

Rubber ferrules.

30

Getting out of a chair and using a walking frame

1

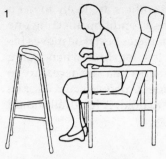

The person shuffles forward to the edge of the seat and, keeping the feet flat on the floor, bends forwards slightly and pushes herself upwards by pressing down on the armrests of the chair.

2

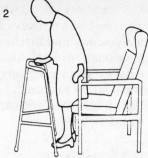

When standing, one hand is transferred to the walking frame, while the other hand remains on the armrest.

3

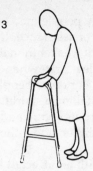

When the person feels secure, both hands are transferred to the walking frame.

Using a walking frame

1
The person places the walking frame approximately 45cm in front of herself.

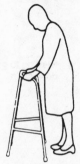

2
When the frame is secure (with all four feet on the ground), she steps into it.

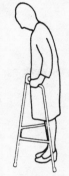

Using a walking frame and getting into a chair

1
The person walks up to the chair.

2
Having reached the chair, she walks round, using the frame for support, until she is in the right position to sit down in the chair.

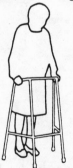

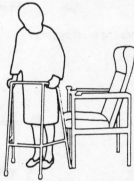

3

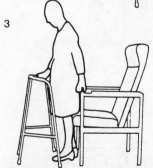

With the frame securely in front of her and calves touching the front of the chair, she puts one hand on an armrest.

4

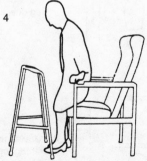

She puts the second hand on the other armrest and lowers herself gently into the chair.

5

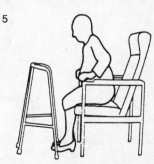

Once in the chair, she can push herself backwards using the support of the armrests.

NOTE: *Some elderly people may need assistance or supervision to perform these activities.*

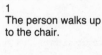
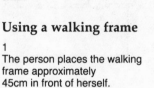

USING STAIRS

Some elderly people may be able to use stairs safely, whilst others are likely to need supervision or assistance. If a person has had a stroke or has a condition affecting one leg, making it weaker than the other, you may find that he manages best if he moves his unaffected leg first when going upstairs and the disabled leg first when going downstairs. For those people who have difficulty in using stairs it may be necessary to consider installing a stairlift or normal lift. In a centre for elderly people stairs *must* be safe, any carpets secure and handrails firmly fixed and easy to hold. A handrail should be fitted at either side if there is sufficient room.

A person with an affected leg using the stairs

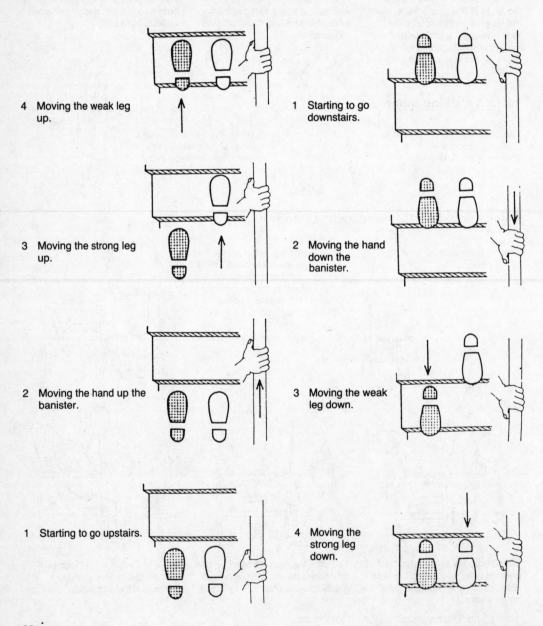

4 Moving the weak leg up.

1 Starting to go downstairs.

3 Moving the strong leg up.

2 Moving the hand down the banister.

2 Moving the hand up the banister.

3 Moving the weak leg down.

1 Starting to go upstairs.

4 Moving the strong leg down.

MOBILITY WITH PEOPLE WHO HAVE SEVERE VISUAL IMPAIRMENT
by Kevin Price

You should speak as you approach a person who is visually impaired, or gently take him by the arm or shoulder and speak to him as you do so. Try not to pull or push him. When you are guiding him along, you should walk one full step in front of him and a little to the side, choosing the side that he prefers. Tell him to place his hand just above your elbow, with his forefingers between your arm and body and his thumb on the outside.

To protect both the upper and lower parts of his body, the person should lift one hand and arm upwards until it is level with his face, with the palm of the hand facing the direction in which he is going. The fingers are spread to give more protection. His hand should be about 20–25cm from his face.

To protect the lower part of his body, he extends his hand forewards and in front of his body, keeping the hand as low as possible and the fingers slightly bent.

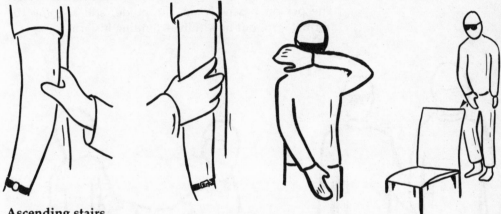

Ascending stairs
If possible, you and the person you are guiding should approach the stairs 'squarely'. You step onto the first stair and wait, showing the person that the level has changed. You may also have to give him instructions.

You ascend the stairs together, the visually impaired person still keeping a grip on you. He can be encouraged to use the banister if he is a little unsure.

On reaching the top of the stairs, you should take one fairly long step forwards to show that you have reached the top and that he has to take only one more step before he is level with you.

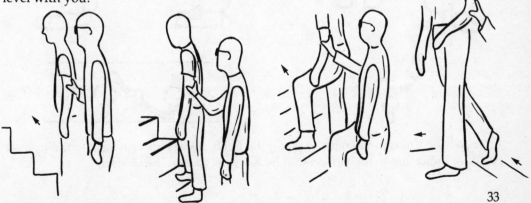

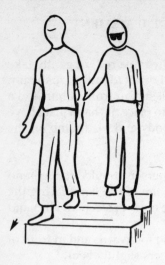

Descending stairs

On reaching the top of the stairs, stop to show the person that the level will change. Walk down one step and encourage the person to find the edge of the top step. He should extend his arm and let you know that he is ready. The two of you descend the stairs together, the person keeping the correct grip on your arm. On reaching the bottom of the stairs, take one fairly long step forwards and wait until the other person has joined you.

Taking a person through a narrow space

In the first drawing, the person is holding on to the guide in the normal way. He is at the guide's side and one pace to the rear. The guide has moved his 'guiding' arm from the side towards the midline of his back and told the person that they are about to go through a narrow place. The person passes *behind* the guide, still keeping the normal grip, but now fully extending his arm.

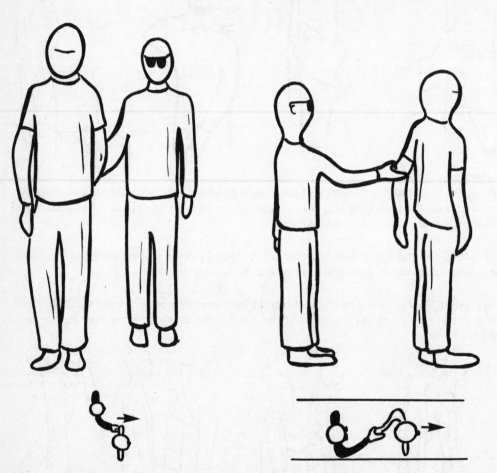

After passing through the narrow place, the guide moves his arm back to the normal position, indicating to the person that he has now passed the obstacle.

34

The different stages in taking a person through a doorway

If possible the person should be on the same side as the door hinges—i.e. on the right side if the door is hinged on the right side. The guide tells the person which way the door opens and how it opens. He holds onto the door handle and allows the visually impaired person to pass his free hand down his arm towards the handle.

In this example, the person is holding onto the right arm of the guide (just above the elbow) with his left hand.

The visually impaired person opens the door, enabling the guide and himself to pass through—the person follows the guide.

The guide and person pass through the doorway—the person pulls the door closed behind him using his free right hand.

NOTE: An elderly person with additional handicaps may need more support.

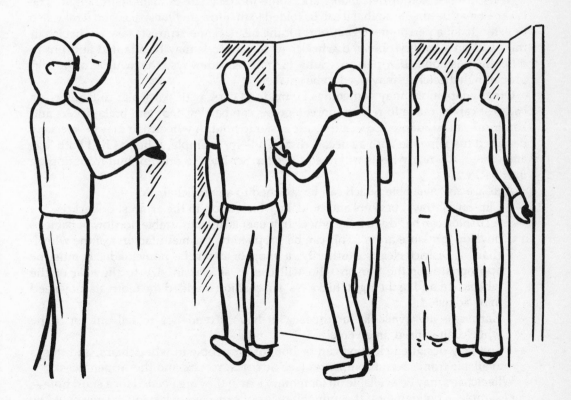

WHEELCHAIRS

If a person has difficulty in moving from one place to another, he may need to use a wheelchair. He may have problems with walking, a tendency to fall, limited or no use of one or both legs; or he may be weak or frail, or have, for example, a heart condition, which could be affected by the exertion of walking.

Wheelchairs are usually provided free by a District Health Authority, although sometimes people prefer to buy their own (a local DHA may be able to advise about this). In the latter case, the cost of maintenance must be borne by the purchaser.

A wheelchair should be suitable for the person who will be using it and should have the adaptations that he needs. Wheelchairs are made in several different ways—they may be folding or rigid, manual or battery-operated, or controlled by the user or an attendant. A rigid wheelchair tends to be more stable, but a folding one is useful if it has to go into the boot of a car or be stored in a confined space. Manual wheelchairs (propelled by hand or pushed from behind) are commonly used, but a battery-operated (electric) one may be more suitable if a person is severely disabled or if the attendant is unable to push a manual wheelchair.

Wheelchairs can be adapted in several ways. The armrests can be fixed if a person is likely to dislodge them, or made removable if someone needs to transfer sideways; the legrests can be fixed or detachable and some footrests are adjustable in height. The backrest may be hinged so that it can be folded to fit into a smaller space, and it may also be extended if a person needs support for the head. Some armrests take a wheelchair tray, and on a battery-operated wheelchair the controls may be adapted and put in different positions. If a person wants to transfer sideways, the wheels on a self-propelling wheelchair may need to be smaller.

Other adaptations may sometimes be made to cope with particular difficulties—a backrest can be made to recline more, legrests can be elevated, and brake levers and handrims can be adapted so that they are easier to hold. A wheelchair may be specially designed for someone with a specific disability—for example, if he has had both legs amputated, the rear wheels will need to be farther back to prevent him from tipping over backwards.

Aids are also available which can be attached to a wheelchair:

— Clip-on ashtrays, beakers and holdalls which fit on to the armrest or backrest.
— A cushion can be added if the wheelchair user is uncomfortable, too low or liable to develop 'pressure areas'. This can be supplied by the manufacturer of the wheelchair, a District Health Authority, a shop or it can be homemade. It must be appropriate for the person who will use it, similar in size to the seat of the wheelchair and of the right thickness. If a cushion is added the footrests may need to be adjusted.
— Harnesses are available for those who have a tendency to fall out, or if the wheelchair is used on a vehicle.
— Specially designed clothing can be bought for people in wheelchairs, and this is available from several companies (see OUTINGS, p. 125, and the Appendices).

Wheelchairs may be available on temporary loan if they are needed for a short time—for example, a holiday, or if the immobility is not expected to last long. They could be provided by a local Social Services or Health Department, or there may be a wheelchair loan scheme in the area. There may be a charge for this service.

Parts of a wheelchair

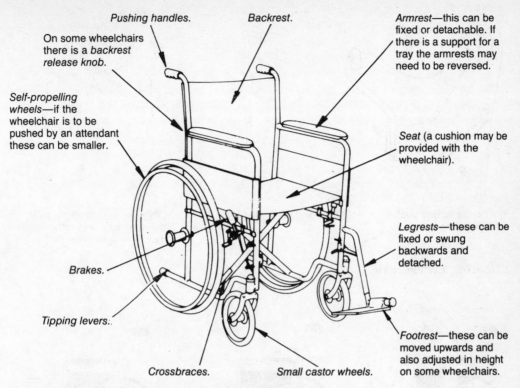

Pushing handles.

On some wheelchairs there is a *backrest release knob.*

Backrest.

Armrest—this can be fixed or detachable. If there is a support for a tray the armrests may need to be reversed.

Self-propelling wheels—if the wheelchair is to be pushed by an attendant these can be smaller.

Seat (a cushion may be provided with the wheelchair).

Brakes.

Legrests—these can be fixed or swung backwards and detached.

Tipping levers:.

Crossbraces.

Small castor wheels.

Footrest—these can be moved upwards and also adjusted in height on some wheelchairs.

(Wheelchairs may vary—the one above was supplied by a DHA.)

Adjusting a wheelchair

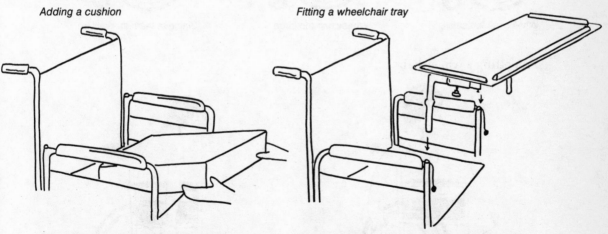

Adding a cushion

Fitting a wheelchair tray

The cushion needs to be the same depth and width as the seat of the wheelchair. Suppliers usually provide cushions which will fit into their wheelchairs—these could be available in different thicknesses. (If a person is incontinent the cover will need to be non-absorbant; if foam is used it must be flame-retardant.)

Fit the armrests so that the tray sockets are at the front of the wheelchair. Remove the toggles and insert the tray.
(The screws underneath the tray may need to be loosened, the position of the tray adjusted and the screws tightened again.)
If a tray cannot be fitted, an attachment may be added to the armrests.

Adjusting a wheelchair *cont*.

Legrests

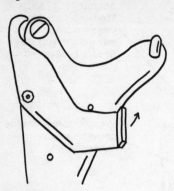 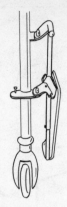 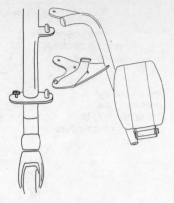

Moving the locking catch to release the legrest.

Swinging the legrest to the side.

Lifting the legrest off the pivot pins to remove it (a retaining pin may have to be taken out).

Choosing a wheelchair

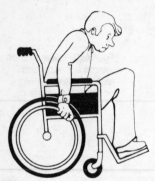 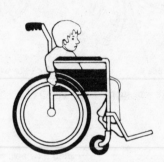 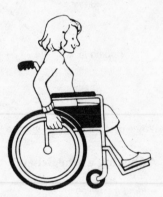

Wheelchair too small.

Wheelchair too large.

Sitting in the right position.

Propelling a wheelchair

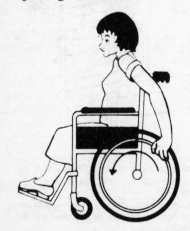 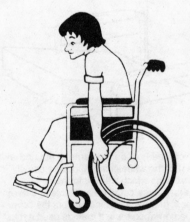

User holding the rim midway at the back and pushing it forward to midway at the front.

User getting into poor position as she pushes from the top of the rim only.

Using a wheelchair

Before taking anyone out in a wheelchair it must be checked to ensure that it is safe, in good working order and not a hazard to someone else. It should be well maintained, have the necessary parts and accessories and be suitable for the user, situation and activity proposed—an electric wheelchair may be designed for indoor or outdoor use.

The elderly user should feel safe and comfortable in the wheelchair and should be able to sit with the hips, knees and ankles at right angles and with the feet flat and secure on the footrests. If he has had a stroke, you will have to watch that his paralysed hand does not fall into the wheels or his affected foot get dragged under the wheelchair. If there is a risk that he might fall out or is travelling in a vehicle, you will have to use a harness. Sometimes elderly people let their arms or hands drop over the edge of the armrests and you should check that these are inside the wheelchair before passing through a narrow space such as a doorway.

If an elderly person is being taken outside he should wear suitable clothing, particularly if it is likely to be cold or if he might have to sit in a draughty area. While pushing a wheelchair you should check that any clothing or rugs do not fall onto the floor or become entangled in the wheels.

The attendant must be trained to handle a wheelchair, look after the person in it and be able to cope should a problem arise. Hazards could include raised threshold strips under doorways, glass doors, steep slopes, ramps without edges, steps, kerbs, potholes, broken pavements, uneven, rough or soft ground, traffic, pedestrians and other people in the centre. If the elderly person is propelling himself he will need to learn how to handle his own wheelchair safely.

Obstacles can often be overcome by pushing down on a tipping lever and easing the wheelchair over them if they cannot be avoided, but some may be quite hazardous—for example, negotiating a flight of steps—and staff need to check that they are trained, able and fit enough to cope with this. Sometimes the elderly person will be able to manage the steps safely, with assistance, or there may be a lift, ramp or subway available.

At least two staff are needed to negotiate steps, and perhaps more if the person is particularly difficult or heavy. It is usually easier if the wheelchair can be taken up and down stairs with the backrest facing the top of the stairs. The helper at the back holds the gripping handles, which should be secure, and the second helper holds the *fixed* struts at the front of the wheelchair. It may be easier to remove the legrests first. The helper at the back needs to be the stronger of the two as he has to take the most strain. If other staff are helping they will need to hold those parts of the wheelchair that are not removable. In all manoeuvres like this staff must remember to bend at the hips and knees and keep their backs straight, not twisted. It helps if someone can act as leader to give instructions. If the wheelchair is electric, the battery may have to be removed beforehand to avoid spillage.

Other points to remember when pushing a wheelchair are: keep it straight if there is a camber in the road or pavement, avoid sudden jerky or fast movements and put both brakes on when the wheelchair is stationary.

A person in a wheelchair usually likes to know what is happening and may want to discuss the details of the journey before it starts. It is also a good idea to tell him about any obstacles or manoeuvres before they happen.

It is important that each elderly person should use his own wheelchair if one has been provided for him. It may have to be marked with his name if it is likely to be used by someone else.

Points to remember
Escalators should be avoided.
Electric wheelchairs should only be used on a pavement except when crossing a road.
Special clothing for people in wheelchairs is available (see OUTINGS, p. 125).

Handling a wheelchair

To open a wheelchair, stand behind the chair and spread the armrests as far apart as possible. With the fingers turned towards the middle of the seat, press downwards with the palms on the supports holding the seat material until the seat is fully opened.

To fold a wheelchair, lift up the footplates and remove the cushion. Stand at the side of the wheelchair and grasp the seat material in the middle, at the front and back, and give a sharp tug upwards. Press the armrests together until the wheelchair is fully closed.

To fold down the backrest, slide down the two backrest release knobs on the backrest and fold down the backrest.
To straighten the backrest, put the backrest into the upright position and pull the knobs upwards (this may not be possible on some wheelchairs).

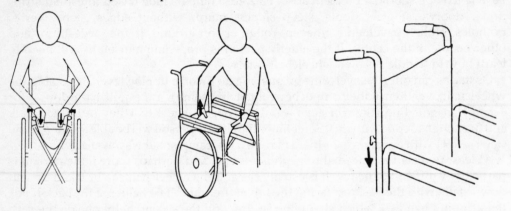

Armrests

Some wheelchairs have detachable armrests which can be released by pulling upwards or by releasing a catch just above the armrest attachment. To replace the armrest, the front part of the armrest is inserted into the front frame socket and then the rear part of the armrest into the back frame socket. When pressed downwards, the armrest may 'click' into place. Detachable armrests may have tray sockets which are used to hold a wheelchair tray. If this is required the armrests are removed and reversed so that the tray socket is at the front of the armrest. Detachable armrests are useful when the elderly person needs to transfer sideways.

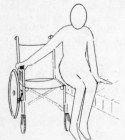

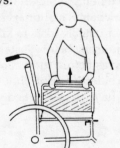

Before lifting the armrest it may be necessary to release a catch underneath.

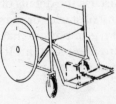

Lifting the footrest.

40

Footplates

These can be pushed to the side to allow a person to get into a wheelchair, and also upwards and downwards, so that the wheelchair user can sit with his hips and knees at right angles. (If a cushion is added to the seat of the wheelchair the footplates are likely to need adjusting again.)

The height of the footplate can be adjusted by loosening and tightening nut 'A' with a spanner. Sometimes also the angle of a footrest can be altered by using a screw attached to the footplate.

Getting in and out of a wheelchair

A wheelchair needs to be used safely or the person in it could fall out or the wheelchair move away.

Both brakes need to be on when a person is getting in or out of a wheelchair—the brake lever may move forwards or backwards depending upon the particular wheelchair. You may have to check how the brakes work from the wheelchair manual.

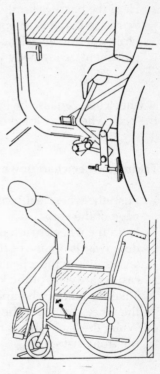

If a person is getting into a wheelchair, ensure that both brakes are on and the footplates hinged upwards so that he can reach the seat. He must *never* stand on the footplates when getting in or out of the wheelchair. (A firm object at the back of the wheelchair, such as a wall or piece of furniture, can make this activity safer.)

To get out of the wheelchair, the user should put on the brakes and hinge the footplates upwards. He holds the armrests and leans forwards slightly, and with both feet firmly on the ground, pushes himself upwards.

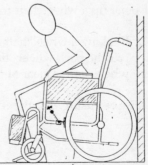

Taking a wheelchair up a kerb

Forwards

1 Push the wheelchair until the footplates are at the edge of the kerb.
2 Holding the handles firmly, push one of the tipping levers down with a foot and tilt the wheelchair backwards until the castors have cleared the kerb.
3 Push the wheelchair forwards until the back wheels touch the kerb, then lower the castors gently onto the pavement.
4 Lift the handles of the wheelchair and push it forward onto the pavement by using the weight of the body.

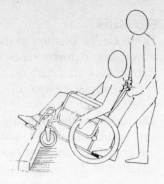

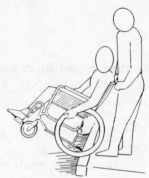

Backwards

1 Bring the wheelchair backwards until the back wheels are touching the edge of the kerb.
2 Hold the handles firmly and tilt the wheelchair backwards so that it is balanced on the back wheels.
3 Firmly lift the wheelchair over the kerb and onto the pavement, using body weight.

A wheelchair can also be lifted backwards onto a pavement by tilting it backwards as the back wheels are lifted over the kerb.

Taking a wheelchair down a kerb

1 Push the wheelchair until the front castors are at the edge of the kerb.
2 Hold the wheelchair handles firmly and press downwards on one of the tipping levers, tilting the wheelchair backwards until the castors are clear of the kerb.
3 Take the foot off the tipping lever and gently lower the wheelchair over the kerb on the back wheels.
4 When the back wheels have cleared the kerb, lower the front castors.

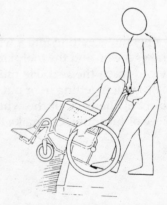

Do *not* tip a wheelchair forwards as the person could fall out.

1 If taking a wheelchair down a kerb backwards, hold the handles firmly and gently roll the back wheels backwards down the kerb. Lower the front castors when the wheelchair is clear of the kerb.

Always ensure that the feet of the elderly person are placed on the footrests.

Taking a wheelchair down a steep slope

This is easier if the wheelchair can be taken down the slope backwards.

Care needs to be taken so that this is not done too quickly.

The occupant of the wheelchair may be able to assist by controlling the propelling wheels or by using the brakes intermittently.

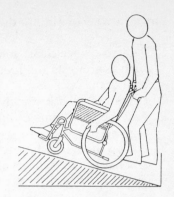

Negotiating a flight of steps

Going upstairs.
Turn the wheelchair until the backrest is facing the stairs, and tilt it until it is balanced. When both attendants are holding it securely, it is 'rolled' up the stairs, one step at a time. Staff may need to reposition themselves after each step. The attendant at the top is two steps above the wheelchair.

Going downstairs. With the wheelchair facing towards the stairs, it is tilted backwards until it is balanced. The attendant in front is three steps below the wheelchair. Holding the wheelchair securely, staff roll it slowly down the stairs one step at a time, repositioning themselves after each step if necessary. To avoid injury, staff need to keep their backs straight, not twisted, and to bend at the hips and knees during the manoeuvre. (It is useful to practise the procedure before using it with elderly people.) One person will need to act as 'leader', giving instructions so that all staff lift simultaneously.

NB. *Carrying a person or a person in a wheelchair up and down stairs should be avoided whenever possible.*

Lifting a wheelchair into the boot of a car

1 Fold the wheelchair, remove any detachable parts such as armrests and footrests, and place near to the boot of the car.

2 Keeping the back straight and hips and knees bent, grip the *fixed* frame of the wheelchair as it is folded together.

3 Lift up the wheelchair vertically, straighten the legs and balance the wheels on the edge of the boot.

4 Tilt the wheelchair towards yourself and, when nearly horizontal, slide the wheelchair into the boot.

5 If the boot varies in width, it may be easier to put the large propelling wheels towards the widest section.

6 Put in any other parts belonging to the chair. A blanket in the boot of the car can sometimes protect the wheelchair and other parts which may move about.

7 If a folded wheelchair is placed in a car in the upright position, it will need to be secured to prevent it from falling over, and both brakes applied to the wheels.

8 When transporting a battery-powered wheelchair, remove the battery and place in the car in an upright position, on a secure flat surface on a piece of newspaper.

Some hazards which may happen when taking a person in a wheelchair on a vehicle lift

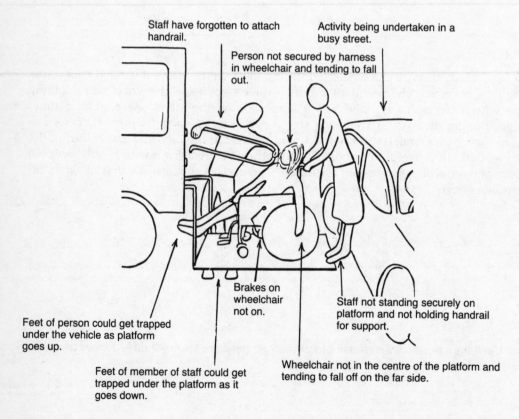

Staff have forgotten to attach handrail.

Activity being undertaken in a busy street.

Person not secured by harness in wheelchair and tending to fall out.

Feet of person could get trapped under the vehicle as platform goes up.

Brakes on wheelchair not on.

Staff not standing securely on platform and not holding handrail for support.

Feet of member of staff could get trapped under the platform as it goes down.

Wheelchair not in the centre of the platform and tending to fall off on the far side.

Maintaining a wheelchair

Wheelchairs need to be cleaned and checked regularly so that they stay in good condition and are safe to use.

Metal parts can be wiped with a damp cloth and later dried; vinyl upholstery can be cleaned with washing-up liquid and warm water—a soft brush may be used on velour material. If a wheelchair tends to become covered with food or with mud from outside, then it is likely to need cleaning more often.

When checking a wheelchair, the following points are particularly important:
* Is the frame bent or damaged?
* Are the tyres worn, soft or cracked?
* Do the brakes work properly against them?
* Are parts of the brakes loose or missing?
* Are any spokes in the wheels faulty?
* Do the castors move freely?
* Is the upholstery worn, torn or damaged?
* Is any of the stitching undone?
* Are any of the straps frayed, worn and insecure?
* Do all the mechanisms work normally?
* Are there loose washers or screws?
* Is a pump available?

Sometimes a wheelchair may be supplied with a toolkit which would include a tyre pressure gauge, pump, screwdriver, pliers, spanners and a puncture repair kit; usually, however, only a pump is provided.

If a wheelchair has been obtained from a District Health Authority it will need to be maintained by an approved repairer except for small repairs. If it has been bought privately, it is worth checking how the repairs should be undertaken and whether the guarantee would be affected by any work done. Often an information manual is supplied with a wheelchair; this usually describes how the wheelchair should be used and serviced. If this is not available or has gone astray, the supplier may provide another copy.

In a centre it is a good idea to have an agreement with a local firm which maintains wheelchairs, so that they can be overhauled at regular intervals and kept in good working order.

NOTE: Batteries for powered wheelchairs should be charged in a well-ventilated room away from anyone who may be smoking or from other people in the room.

Tyres

Tyres need to be firm enough for the brakes to hold and for the wheelchair not to slip. Wheelchair tyres may have one of two types of valve, a 'Woods' type or a 'Schrader' type. When pumping up a tyre with a 'Woods' type valve, an additional piece must be screwed onto the connection on the pump. The recommended tyre pressure for inflatable tyres may be marked on the tyre. If the tyre pressure is lost from the 'Woods' valve, check that cap A is tight (see diagram).

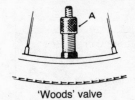 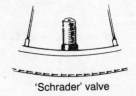 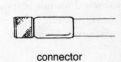

'Woods' valve   'Schrader' valve   adaptor   connector

Repairing a wheelchair

Problem	Cause	Action
Brakes not working very well.	1 Brake and tyre not making proper contact.	Pump up tyres to correct pressure, or check correct pressure on powered chair. (NB: Do not use air line at a local garage unless recommended by the supplier.)
	2 Brake fittings may have become loose.	Reposition and tighten using a screwdriver or spanner.
Puncture.	Damage to the tyre and/ or inner tube.	Replace the tyre or inner tube.
No puncture evident but soft ride and tyres need pumping up very frequently.	A valve may be leaking.	Replace the valve or inner tube (supplier or a bicycle shop may be able to help).
Wheelchair pulls to one side on a level surface.	1 Front castor on that side may require adjustment.	Check that the castor swings freely. If you cannot adjust it yourself, ask the supplier for help.
	2 Tyres may be low on that side.	Pump them up.
Handrims are loose and wobbly.	Probably due to general wear and tear or prolonged use.	Tighten the rims using a spanner or screwdriver.
Spokes are loose.	Probably due to general wear and tear or prolonged use.	Tighten or replace. (Bicycle shop may be able to help if necessary.)
Footrests are loose and uncomfortable.	Probably due to general wear and tear or prolonged use.	Readjust and tighten using a spanner or screwdriver. Correctly adjusted footrests contribute to comfort.
Frame bent.	Most commonly happens to manual wheelchairs when they are stored in a boot of a car and other heavy items are stored on top of them.	If the damage is slight you may be able to rectify it yourself taking care not to cause further damage. Do not hit it with a heavy object. If in doubt consult the supplier as the strength of the frame can be affected even by small dents.
Chair is stiff and difficult to manoeuvre.	Movable parts seizing up.	Oil at the points indicated by the supplier.
Battery not recharging when plugged in.	Plug and/or socket connections may have shaken loose whilst the chair is in use.	Check the plug and socket. Check fuse and reset button if there is one.
Chair does not respond to commands even after charging the battery.	1 Circuit breaker may have tripped.	Reset the circuit breaker.
	2 Charger may still be plugged into chair.	Disconnect the charger.

The above chart is taken from the book *Choosing a Wheelchair* published by RADAR.

4 LIFTING AND MOVING ELDERLY PEOPLE

Before an elderly person is moved or lifted, staff must have some understanding of lifting methods and know which one to use in each case. They will have to decide whether it can be done by one person or by more and whether any equipment may be needed.

They need to know how to hold the person's body in a good position that will prevent back injuries to themselves, other staff or the person being lifted, and they must also be secure enough to control the lift safely. Different lifts may be done with the same elderly person at different times, depending on his ability, co-operation and condition, and on the particular situation.

Before doing the lift the elderly person should be assessed: Is he able to help with the lift? What is his condition? Is he able to take his own weight? Is he alert and co-operative? Is he heavy or large? And so on.

The kind of lift has to be decided and which staff can do it. Someone needs to act as leader to give instructions if more than one member of staff is taking part in it. Everyone should be in the right position—for example, with the feet apart, back straight and untwisted, hips and knees bent and grasping each other or the elderly person securely. After the instruction 'One, two, three and lift', staff lift together, straightening their legs if necessary until the person is moved to another position.

If a person is able, it may be possible for him to transfer sideways out of a wheelchair or to use an aid for support.

Many books have been written on lifting and handling people. These are worth reading, but perhaps one of the best ways of learning is to attend a course run by an experienced person who is able to teach and demonstrate the different techniques and enable staff to try out the lifts for themselves. It is important to practise the lifts before starting to use them unsupervised.

Courses on lifting and handling may be organised locally or nationally by a Health or Social Services department, a physiotherapy unit or another group, and it is wise to ask around if there is no one in the centre who is able to run one.

As equipment and procedures may change from time to time, it is important to keep up to date and be aware of any new methods which may be easier and safer to use.

Lifting or moving people or loads

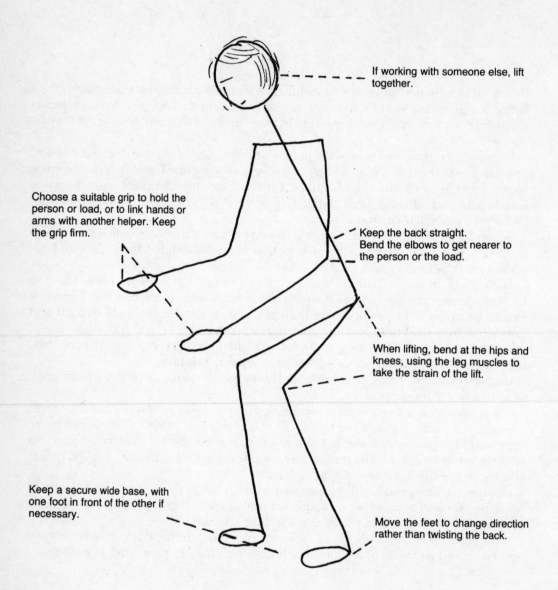

If working with someone else, lift together.

Choose a suitable grip to hold the person or load, or to link hands or arms with another helper. Keep the grip firm.

Keep the back straight. Bend the elbows to get nearer to the person or the load.

When lifting, bend at the hips and knees, using the leg muscles to take the strain of the lift.

Keep a secure wide base, with one foot in front of the other if necessary.

Move the feet to change direction rather than twisting the back.

Some points which may need to be considered before lifting an elderly person

Am I fit and able enough to handle this person?

Am I wearing suitable clothing, such as non-slip shoes?

Have I explained clearly to the elderly person what I am about to do and how he can co-operate? Is any equipment readily available?

Do I know the principles of lifting?

Has his condition or mood changed? Can I use the same lift I used previously?

Please, Miss, can I sit in another chair?

How much can the elderly person do for himself?

Is the elderly person too heavy or awkward to lift? Would a hoist be more suitable?

What shall I need to do to assist him?

How many staff will be needed to perform the lift? Who will be in charge?

Which type of lift shall I need to use?

Have I been shown and practised the lift I am about to use?

Can I do it on my own or shall I need help?

49

5 COMMUNICATION

COMMUNICATION PROBLEMS IN ELDERLY PEOPLE
by Isobel O'Leary

There are various reasons why elderly people may have difficulty with communication. Some of the conditions which affect their ability are quite common, including deafness, blindness and general lack of stimulation. However, there are also certain medical conditions that impair communication, such as Parkinson's disease, motor neurone disease (MND), multiple sclerosis (MS), dementia, depression and, perhaps most importantly, strokes.

The distinction between 'speech' and 'communication' is important. The latter includes speech, but also takes in facial expressions, hand movements, reading and writing, as well as the ability to understand other people's communication.

In Parkinson's disease, motor neurone disease and multiple sclerosis, the main communication problem is with speaking, since these diseases cause difficulty in the physical production of sounds and words, due to weakness or lack of co-ordination of the speech muscles. This problem is called *dysarthria*, and results in speech that may sound slurred, very quiet, monotonous or jerky.

Communication problems after a stroke

A stroke causes some damage to the brain. If this occurs in the part of the brain that controls the ability to deal with language, the person will probably suffer from a condition called *dysphasia*. The language area for most people is in the left side of the brain, so dysphasia often occurs with a right hemiplegia, since the left side of the brain affects the right side of the body. Many dysphasic people have difficulties in understanding (receptive dysphasia) and in formulating language (expressive dysphasia), whether it is spoken or written. Each person's communication problems are different and what helps one person may not help another.

People with receptive dysphasia

Elderly people with this problem may have difficulty in understanding other people's speech or written material. They often appear to be understanding more than they actually can. This is because it is a distressing condition to suffer and the person may try to cover up his disability, but he may also get clues to what you are saying from your facial expression, hand movements, tone of voice or the context of the conversation; in addition, although he may only understand a few words, he may be able to follow the gist of the conversation without being able to grasp specific instructions.

Even when people have receptive difficulties, do not talk down to them or raise your voice. If their hearing and intellect are intact this approach will only increase their frustration. However, do try to simplify what you are saying, slow down and do not be afraid to repeat things. Make sure that the person has understood you. Many people will find that noise, tiredness or upset will affect their concentration and their ability to understand.

People with expressive dysphasia

With this problem people have difficulty in using spoken or written language and nearly always suffer from feelings of frustration. Often a person will know what he wants to say, but is unable to find the words. He may also make mistakes in his use of language—for example, he may say 'soap' when he means 'towel', he may produce jargon or meaningless words such as 'histar', or he may make incorrect sounds within words, such as 'ken' when he means 'pen'. He may also use the words 'yes' and 'no' inappropriately. He may use words and phrases repetitively, as if he is unable to break away from the word he keeps saying, such as a swear word, or he may produce a flow of meaningless speech which he does not try to stop—this usually means that he is unaware that it does not make sense.

Do not make such a person feel rushed. He often needs time to grasp what you are saying and to formulate what he wants to say in reply. It may be helpful if you communicate with him by gesture. Encourage a person when he is making an effort to talk. Make him feel confident so that he will try to communicate, for he probably feels embarrassed by his speech difficulty.

People with dyspraxia

Following a stroke a person may suffer from an additional problem called *dyspraxia*. This is an inability to produce voluntary muscle movements, despite adequate muscle function. For example, a person may smile at you in greeting, but be unable to smile when specifically asked to do so. He may have difficulty in making movements in the right order, and this is often worst when he is trying to start the movement; once he has got going, the movement may be reasonable. Dyspraxia can affect the limbs as well as the speech muscles, so that eating or dressing may be unco-ordinated. Even when there is actual muscle weakness, as often happens after a stroke, it is not enough to explain the mistakes that happen.

Typically, a person with dyspraxia has slow and laboured speech, but some words may pop out easily, such as 'I'm all right' or 'Hello'. He is often unaware of errors and may become frustrated at the lack of voluntary control over the articulatory muscles. He may make frequent repeats and attempts at self-correction.

All the conditions outlined above have different effects on a person's speech and general communication. Sometimes the cause of the problem is not clear—for example, it may be difficult to decide whether a person's failure to speak or communicate in any way is due to the effects of the stroke, or whether it is because he is depressed and withdrawn, or both. Slurred dysarthric speech occurs with several diseases, as I have mentioned, and can also occur after a stroke. When an elderly person uses a lot of apparently meaningless speech, staff need to establish whether it is due to confusion, dementia or the specific language problem of dysphasia. A speech and language therapist will be able to give advice on the most helpful approach for each particular person.

Definitions of words you may hear

Dysphasia: difficulty in understanding and/or using language.

Dysarthria: difficulty with the physical production of sounds and words due to muscle weakness or lack of co-ordination.

Dyspraxia: inability to produce voluntary muscle movements despite adequate muscle function.

Dysphagia: (not to be confused with *dysphasia*) difficulty in swallowing.

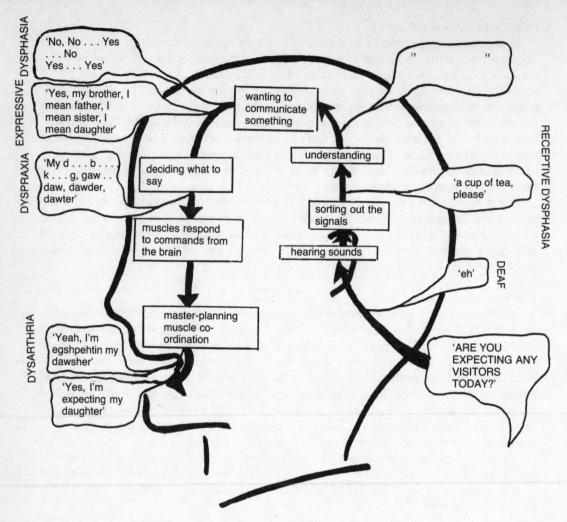

Diagrammatic view of the brain and different speech problems

HEARING AIDS
by Elizabeth Highfield

Hearing loss may be slight or severe and its cause can be divided into two main categories:

1 *Conductive hearing loss*. When the outer or middle ear has been affected, this type of hearing loss is often treatable.
2 *Sensori-neural loss*. This is caused when the nerves within the inner ear have been affected. It is an untreatable condition and is the most common cause of hearing loss in elderly people. As a result, many elderly people with hearing impairment are fitted with a hearing aid.

Types of hearing aid
1 *Behind the ear hearing aids*
   These are worn behind the ear and are connected to earmoulds by a piece of plastic tubing. To fit the aid, place the earmould into the ear first, then hook the aid over the top of the ear, placing it behind. If glasses are worn, put these on first with the aid

outside, between the glasses and the ear. The majority of patients wear this type of hearing aid.

2 *Body worn hearing aids*
These are rarely issued today—only usually to those patients who have a profound hearing loss. This type of aid has a 'box' which fits onto clothing, with a wire connecting the box to a small earphone with earmould attached.

Maintenance
Occasionally the hearing aid may develop a slight fault. The table below lists some common faults and solutions.

HEARING AID FAULT FINDING TABLE

Problem	Check	Fault	Solution
Aid dead	Tubing	Condensation in tube	Remove earmould and blow out
	Earmould	Earmould blocked with wax	Remove earmould and clean
	Battery	Battery flat, wrong way round	Examine, test and replace
Buzzing noise	On/off switch	Switch on 'T'	Reset switch to 'M'
		Microphone broken	Return for repair
Crackling intermittent problems	Battery contacts switch volume control	Faulty connections	Return hearing aid to Hearing Aid Services for repair
Whistling	Earmould	a) Poorly fitting mould b) Incorrect mould insertion.	Check earmould fit Return to Hearing Aid Service for replacement tube or earmould.
	Tubing	Hole in tubing	
	Ear canal	Wax	Refer to GP

Note: On a hearing aid the following letters may be marked:
  'O' = Off
  'M' = Microphone (on)
  'T' = for use with a telephone, television or loop system

Earmoulds
These are individually moulded and must be a perfect fit to avoid soreness or feedback (whistling). The earmould should be cleaned daily by removing the mould from the hearing aid and washing it in warm soapy water. DO NOT USE A DETERGENT.

How to obtain an NHS hearing aid

Anyone who wishes to try an NHS aid must be referred by their general practitioner to the local Hearing Aid Services Department for hearing assessment. Some areas may still be referring patients to the local ENT Department.

If a hearing aid is issued by the local hospital it will be maintained free of charge and replaced when necessary. If the aid has been purchased from a private supplier it is likely that it will need to be returned to the supplier for repair and that a charge will be made for the work done.

Environmental aids for hearing impaired people

These devices are supplementary to using a hearing aid and are designed to assist in specific areas. Depending on the locality, these aids may be available through the NHS or Social Services. However, all these devices can be purchased from numerous retail outlets.

1 *Television Aids.* A portable personal system for listening to the television with an independent volume control.
2 *Telephone adaptors.* These can assist with:
   a) Amplification of ring tone—extra loud bell.
                              —variability of type of ring.
   b) Amplification of voice   —speech amplifier volume control.
                              —inductive coupler to be used only in conjunction with the 'T' position of a hearing aid.
3 *Doorbell.* Frequently, hearing impaired patients may be unaware of callers but can be helped by:
   a) Extra loud doorbell.
   b) A flashing light. The doorbell is connected to either a single light (for example, in the living room), or to all the lights in the house, with adaptation for day or night usage.

When an elderly person is first issued with a hearing aid, he or she may find the background noises very distracting, so it is recommended that the aid should be used only at home for the first few weeks. Once the user has become more confident, he can try the hearing aid outside, but traffic noises can appear to be quite loud. It should be noted that it can take up to three months or more to get the full benefit from the hearing aid.

Many Social Services Departments employ social workers for the deaf, or other staff who are able to give advice about aids and equipment and can also suggest services which may be available for hearing impaired people in the area. Local hospital departments, too, may have the service of volunteers who visit hearing impaired people to give advice about hearing aids and so on. If you encounter problems with hearing aids or other equipment and need information, it may be helpful to contact the local Hearing Aid Services Department who will be happy to advise you.

Batteries

All hearing aids use a battery which will need to be replaced at regular intervals. The length of time the battery will last depends on how powerful the hearing aid is. Supplies of batteries for NHS hearing aids can be obtained from the local Hearing Aid Services Department free of charge; however, if the aid has been purchased privately, supplies will have to be bought from a local retail outlet.

The Golden Rules of good communication with hearing impaired people
For those who have hearing impairment, clear speech, body language and facial expression are essential as an aid to understanding the spoken word. The following actions on your part will assist in communication:

1 Be patient.
2 Attract the person's attention before speaking.
3 Keep your face visible and ensure that it is well lit; remember not to hide your mouth with your hands.
4 Always look at the person you are speaking to.
5 Do not shout. Speak clearly and not too quickly.
6 Do not break your rhythm when speaking. Lip-reading is usually in phrases, not in words.
7 Do not keep repeating the same phrase if not initially understood—change your wording.
8 Remember to write down important information such as the date of the next appointment, or when and how medication should be taken.
9 Remember that a hearing aid amplifies background noise as well as speech.
10 Use your hands in gesture whenever practical to do so.

Why does a hearing aid whistle?
Whistling happens when the sound produced by the hearing aid feeds back into the microphone. Normally a hearing aid should not whistle when it is being worn; if it does, there may be various causes.

Is the earmould properly in the ear?
Quite often the user fails to insert the top point of the mould properly. This is like expecting false teeth to work when they are not correctly in place.
   If the mould is not a *good fit* it may need replacing. This will be carried out by the Hearing Aid Services Department.

Is the volume too high?
If the hearing aid volume wheel is set at its maximum it is likely to whistle. A stronger hearing aid may be needed.

Is there ear wax or any other blockage in the meatus (ear channel)?
Consult with the GP if this is thought to be the problem.

Is the tube cracked?
A hole or crack in the tube that leads to the hearing aid will cause whistling. The Hearing Aid Services Department or sometimes the patient himself will replace the tubing.

Is the earmould or tube blocked?
Condensation or wax can block the tube. Remove the obstruction.

PART TWO

ACTIVITIES

INTRODUCTION

Before giving an elderly person an activity, find out whether he already has any interests, which he enjoys most and whether he would like to try anything new. Aids can often be provided if someone has difficulty in doing an activity, and sometimes it can be done in a different way if this makes it easier.

In the following pages the activities have been divided into craftwork, games and other activities. There are of course many other activities that elderly people can do, but those included may stimulate further ideas.

If an elderly person has a disability or a condition that could be affected by taking part in an activity, you should make sure that what you are proposing is suitable for him— for example, it would be unwise to suggest a strenuous activity for someone who has a serious heart condition, or to put someone who is liable to have fits, bouts of unconsciousness or dizziness in a situation where there are obstacles, furniture or equipment that could be a hazard if an accident occurred. People with respiratory conditions should be discouraged from attempting activities that are dusty or could give off fumes, vapours or particles into the air; this might happen if someone were sanding a piece of wood or using certain kinds of wool.

When doing an activity, the elderly person should be in the most comfortable position for the job in hand—either sitting upright with the hips, knees and ankles at a right angle or standing at a table which has been adjusted to the right height. If he is sitting in a chair, this may need to have a backrest and arms so that it gives him more support and prevents him from falling out easily (see also STROKE, p. 20).

Any activity given to an elderly person should be safe for him to do; he should not be at risk of harming himself, anyone else or of damaging property. It is a good idea for people to have their own tools and materials and to keep these in a container for their own use. This could be a box, or a bag which can be hung on the back of a wheelchair or locker. Each box or bag could be labelled with the owner's name, so that it would not get lost or be used by someone else.

Sometimes activities have to fit in with the running of the centre—either because the main purpose of the centre is the nursing and care of the elderly people, or because there may be a limited number of staff available. It may therefore be more convenient to provide craftwork in the mornings, for those who can manage without a lot of help, and to organise social activities in the afternoons when more staff may be available. If any other services are provided, such as physiotherapy, occupational therapy, chiropody, social work or hairdressing, arrangements for activities will have to be organised around these, too.

In a residential centre it may be possible to plan activities around a timetable— dominoes on a Monday afternoon, bingo on Tuesday and Thursday afternoons, a whist drive on a Wednesday afternoon and table games on a Friday afternoon. In a day centre these activities may need to be staggered if people attend on the same days each week. Other events programmed into the timetable could be a service on alternate Sundays and a social on the first Tuesday of the month. There could also be special events, such as a birthday celebration, an Easter Bonnet parade, Harvest Festival, a bazaar, exhibition or sale of work, and a jumble sale. All these add interest and give the elderly people something to look forward to. Projects such as fund-raising for a minibus can also give a sense of purpose.

Most activities can normally be undertaken in a day room or lounge, although some, like snooker and baking, are best done in another area. In some centres, different rooms are used for different purposes—a TV room, a reading room, a quiet room, a games room and so on—and this can be useful in a long-stay unit where the residents may have to stay in the same room with the same people over a long period of time.

If there are no staff to provide activities, it may be possible to use the television and radio as a source of entertainment, and also a music centre which can be used to play records, discs and tapes chosen by the elderly people.

When trying to encourage elderly people to join in an activity, they should never be made to take part against their will, although often a little persuasion is required.

If you have difficulty in obtaining any of the equipment and materials mentioned in the following pages, please refer to the names and addresses of suppliers listed in the appendices.

6 CRAFTWORK

ART

In a centre art can provide opportunities for interesting and creative activity for those who are unable to attempt anything more strenuous. Work can be fixed to a table with sellotape, Blu-tac or drawing board clips, or it can be pinned to a board which is placed on a non-slip surface. Pencils and brushes can be built up with padding (or Rubazote) if they are too slender to hold, or extra-large brushes can be bought.

If a person is unable to draw but enjoys painting, it may be possible to buy sketches on paper or board from the local art shop which may also supply 'art kits' containing instructions and all necessary materials. Some elderly people may find these a little difficult and may prefer to do a 'painting by numbers' picture which can be bought at a local toy shop. If you have difficulty obtaining these, a print shop may be able to photocopy drawings onto art paper, or you could trace them onto art paper or board using tracing or greaseproof paper.

In some centres there may be equipment to make drawing and painting easier—easels, water pots and paint pots that can be secured, and a good supply of art paper, sketch pads, brushes and paints for watercolour and oil painting—while in others items may need to be purchased as they are needed.

Some elderly people have a tendency to knock over paint pots or water jars and you may have to provide containers that are easier for them to use—a large, flat-bottomed ashtray is excellent for holding water and supporting brushes—or you could use a double suction aid to secure containers. A water pot is available that holds brushes and has a lid to prevent spillage of water. It can also be completely closed when not in use.

NOTE: *Cleaning brushes*. Brushes used for oil paint can be rinsed in white spirit and then washed with soap; brushes used for watercolours can be rinsed in cold water, while those used for acrylic paint can be washed with cold water and soap. If acrylic paint or oil paint has dried on a brush, it can be softened with paint solvent, cleaned as above and stored upside down in a jar.

A CHAMOIS LEATHER RING

Threading chamois leather pieces onto a strip of nylon offcut (nytrim) can be a popular activity with elderly people as it is easy to do, even by someone with quite limited abilities. Care needs to be taken to ensure that a person is safe in using a bodkin and that it is not too sharp. A member of staff can make holes in the chamois leather pieces, although there may be an elderly person who can do it safely.

Securing the bodkin

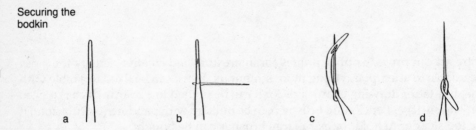

a) Trim end 7.5–10cm of the nytrim until only 4–7mm wide. Make a slit in the middle. b) Thread on the bodkin. c) Insert the bodkin through the slit and pull through. d) Tighten.

Cut small pieces of chamois leather about 4cm across from the larger pieces. Pierce the centre of each piece over a spike (use a long rustproof nail hammered through a sanded piece of wood about 11.5cm sq. and 2cm deep clamped to a table.

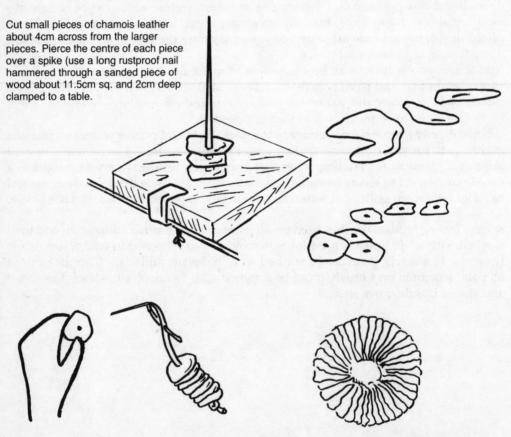

Thread the pieces onto a strip of nytrim about 40cm long with a knot at one end, until the length of the chamois pieces is 25cm when pushed together.

Release the bodkin and then tie the two ends together firmly and securely with a non-slip knot. Trim the ring with scissors.

CROCHET

Crochet is a simple and interesting craft which can be done by elderly people while they are talking to their friends.

It is built up on a series of chain stitches which can be used to create different patterns and designs. At first, very little is needed except a crochet hook, a pattern and some yarn (crochet cotton, nylon strip or wool, though other yarns can also be used).

Crochet hooks can be bought in a variety of sizes and chosen to suit the yarn being used—generally the thicker the yarn, the larger the hook. Very thick crochet hooks can be used by elderly people who may have some difficulty with sight or in using finer hooks. Dark or chunky yarn is also easier to see.

Patterns can sometimes be obtained in large print, or ordinary patterns can be 'blown up' on a photocopying machine. If these are kept in a polythene sleeve, the pattern stays clean for the next person and it can also be kept in a file for later use.

Craft booklets can be bought in local shops, giving a variety of simple patterns which can be made in quite a short time.

Method

1
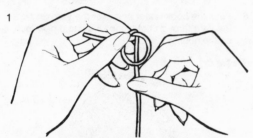
Hold yarn between the thumb and forefinger of left hand. Form a loop with the other hand.

2
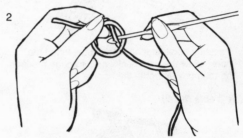
Draw the yarn through the loop with a crochet hook.

3
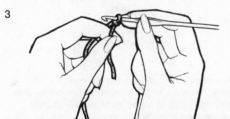
Keeping the hook in the loop, pull the knot together.

4
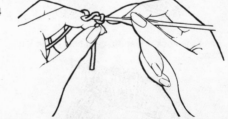
Pass yarn around little finger, across palm and behind forefinger of left hand. Hold the hook in right hand. Pull yarn gently so that it lies firmly around the fingers.

5
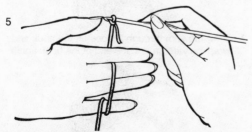
Hold short end of yarn between thumb and forefinger of left hand.

6
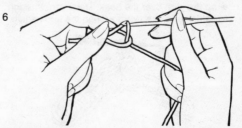
Pass the hook under the yarn and draw backwards through the loop.

Chain(ch)

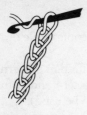 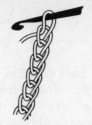

1 After making a slip knot on the hook, pass the hook under and over the yarn and bring the yarn back through the loop.

2 Using the new loop, pass the hook under and over the yarn and bring backwards.

Slip Stitch(ss)

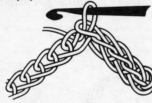

1 Pass the hook into the stitch to the left of the hook, draw the yarn backwards through the loop on the hook and onto the hook.

Half Treble (hlf tr)

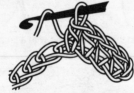

1 Pass the hook under the yarn held in the left hand.

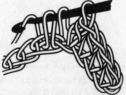

2 Insert the hook through 3rd stitch on the left, wrap the yarn over the hook. Draw yarn through the stitch and wrap yarn around the hook again.

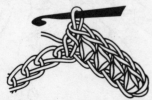

3 Draw the yarn through all the loops on the hook leaving a new loop.

Double Crochet(dc)

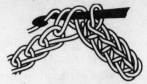

1 Pass the hook into the second stitch on the left.

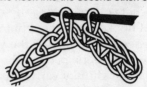

2 Draw the yarn through the stitch leaving two loops on the hook.

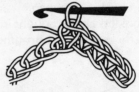

3 Pass the hook under and over the yarn and draw the yarn through both loops leaving a new loop on the hook.

Treble (tr)

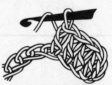

1 Pass the hook under the yarn in the left hand.

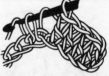

2 Insert the hook into the 4th stitch on the left, pass hook under the yarn and draw backwards through stitch (3 loops on hook). Wrap yarn around the hook again.

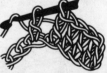

3 Draw the yarn through 2 loops on the hook and wrap the yarn around the end of the hook again.

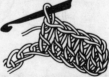

4 Draw the yarn through last 2 loops leaving a new loop on the hook.

EMBROIDERY

This can be an enjoyable pastime for those who have plenty of time to spare and have full use of their fingers and hands. It can be quite easy when using simple stitches and transfered cloths or it may be more complicated.

Most materials are fairly easy to obtain, although the kits can be expensive and you may need to economise by making up your own kits and using transfers. Material with a larger weave, such as Binca, is particularly useful for those who are unable to see fine work clearly, and the *coton à broderie* cottons are easy to use with the larger bodkins. Sometimes the stranded cotton needs to be split.

If people have the use of only one hand they may welcome an embroidery frame with a clamp or on a stand, or they may prefer to stitch their work onto a standing tapestry frame. Needles can be threaded by inserting them into a firm pincushion for support and needle threaders can make the threading easier. Self-threading needles with an open end are also available (see SEWING, p. 87).

Magnifiers can be bought which hang round the neck and these are ideal for elderly people who want to see the work more clearly while keeping both hands free.

Nottingham Rehab supply stirex scissors with an easy-cut action, and items such as pins with heads, left-handed scissors, and pin boxes with clips or suction cups are available from needlework shops.

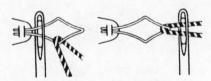

Using a needle threader to pass thread through a needle.

An aid to hold an embroidery cloth

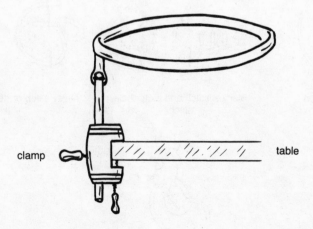

clamp   table

The ring can be fixed at any angle to suit the individual and is useful for a person with the use of only one hand.

Some embroidery stitches

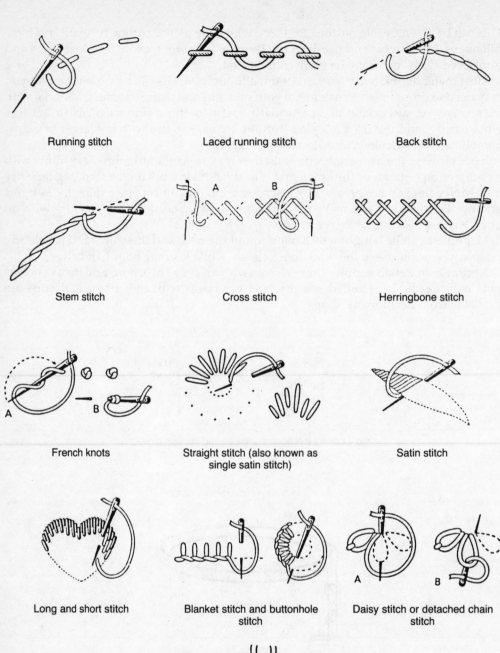

Running stitch

Laced running stitch

Back stitch

Stem stitch

Cross stitch

Herringbone stitch

French knots

Straight stitch (also known as single satin stitch)

Satin stitch

Long and short stitch

Blanket stitch and buttonhole stitch

Daisy stitch or detached chain stitch

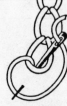

Chain stitch

GIFT TAGS, CALENDARS AND CARDS

Items like these are usually cheap to make and are within the capabilities of many elderly people. All that is needed is a selection of used birthday or Christmas cards, some thin coloured string, a paper punch, glue for paper, ribbon, small cellophane or polythene bags, some fairly thick sheets of card for the calendars (already cut if possible), pieces of thinner card for the greetings cards (cut to size) and some small calendars.

Gift tags

These can be made from used Christmas or birthday cards or any other suitable pictures on strong enough card. The picture on the card must be appropriate—half a candle or an incomplete scene will not do. The picture can be cut out with normal scissors or pinking shears but needs to be cut cleanly and in a straight line if it is a square tag. If pinking shears are used, each cut must match the previous one. Tags can be any size, but 7×7cm has been found to be a good size. If the tags are to be folded down the centre they will need to be a little longer—13×7cm.

When the tag has been cut, a hole is punched in the top left-hand corner with a punch and a piece of string threaded through it. If the tags are being made to raise funds, a small number can be placed in a transparent bag, sealed and sold.

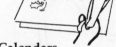
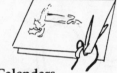

Calendars

This is another useful idea which can also be used to raise funds just before Christmas. An attractive picture can be cut from a birthday or Christmas card and stuck on the upper half of a fairly thick piece of card. These are sometimes available already cut from stationers; otherwise a large sheet will have to be cut to the right size. When cutting by hand, the desired size of the calendar (e.g. 23×15cm) should be ruled in pencil as a guide. If the card is very thick, a sharp craft knife and metal rule may be needed to cut it, and the card should be cut on a board to protect the table.

A small calendar is glued onto the lower part of the card and a piece of ribbon about 10cm long onto the top of the card at the back. A small stick-on label can be used to cover the glued ends of ribbon.

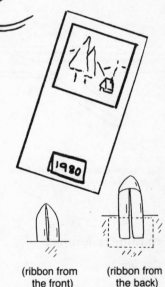

(ribbon from the front) (ribbon from the back)

Cards

Interesting features can be cut out of pictures and glued onto folded pieces of card to make new greetings cards.

Glues

Uhu or a similar all-purpose glue can be used for sticking the ribbon. For sticking paper, elderly people will find PrittStick easy to use.

KNITTING

Many elderly people, particularly women, have done knitting before and will happily work at it while talking to friends. The scope for the craft is very wide—from simple dishcloths, pot-holders, scarves and covers for coat-hangers and so on, to quite intricate garments. Those who have been knitting for years and can still do so will be able to complete the work unaided; others may have some difficulty and may need aids to make the activity easier. Larger knitting needles, thicker wool, row counters and large print knitting patterns will all help here. If someone finds two knitting needles hard to hold, she may manage better with a circular needle. For those who only have the use of one hand there are several aids which support a knitting needle, as well as knitting frames and machines. Some people may even like to try French knitting, using a wooden bobbin: the kits can be bought from craft and toy shops.

Knitting is normally done right-handed—the stitch is worked onto the right needle—but some people may find it easier to work left-handed, working the stitch onto the left-hand needle.

One of the great advantages of knitting is that it can be continued at home by those who attend a day centre. This is particularly beneficial if they can no longer pursue their former interests, and live alone.

Stitching seams

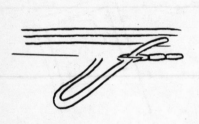

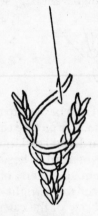

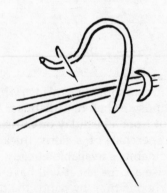

Backstitch is a secure stitch for a strong seam.

Stitch which can be used to make an invisible seam.

Overstitch is a useful stitch for joining ribbed knitting together.

Knitting techniques

Casting on

Knot a loop at the end of the yarn—pass onto left-hand pin.

Pass the yarn under and over the right-hand pin.

Draw the right-hand pin backwards . . .

Knitting techniques *cont.*

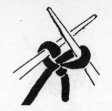

. . . until another loop is formed.

Slip the new loop onto the left-hand pin.

Insert the right-hand pin between the new stitches to make the next stitch.

Knit stitch

Pass the right-hand pin through the stitch on the left-hand pin.

Pass the yarn over the end of the right-hand pin.

Draw the yarn towards the stitch and bring right-hand pin backwards.

Bring the right-hand pin upwards.

Slip over the other pin.

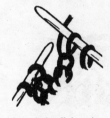

Slide the stitch off the pin.

Purl stitch

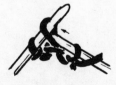

Slip the right-hand pin through the front of the next stitch.

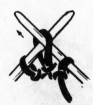

Push the pin forwards.

Wrap the yarn around the end of the right-hand pin.

Draw the yarn downwards and bring the pin with it.

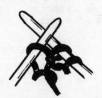

Slip the right-hand pin through the loop on the left-hand pin.

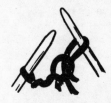

Slip the stitch off the left-hand pin.

69

Knitting techniques *cont.*

Casting off

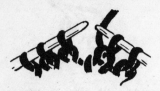

Knit two stitches.

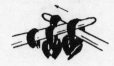

Slip first stitch over second stitch.

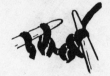

Knit the next stitch and pass the stitch on the right-hand pin over this stitch. Continue until casting-off is complete.

Picking up dropped stitches

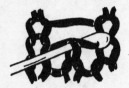
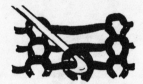

Picking up 'dropped' stitches on the knit side—on the purl side.

Two ways of increasing in knitting

A

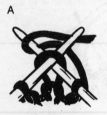
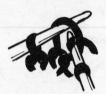
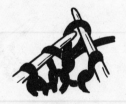
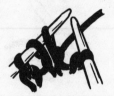

Pass the right-hand pin through the next stitch—slip the yarn over the end.

Bring the loop backwards.

Slip the loop onto the left-hand pin.

Knit the new stitch.

B

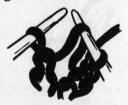
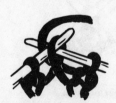

Pick up the yarn between the two stitches.

Twist and slip the yarn onto the left-hand pin. Knit the new stitch.

70

Two ways of decreasing in knitting

A

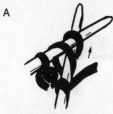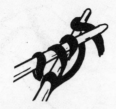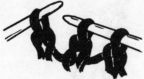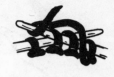

Push right-hand pin into next two stitches on left-hand pin.

Pass yarn over right-hand pin in normal way.

Slip the two stitches off the pin to form one stitch.

Decreasing in purl stitch.

B

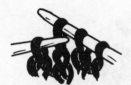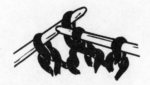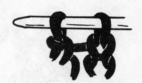

Knit two stitches in the normal way.

Slip the first stitch over the second stitch.

Slip the first stitch off the pin.

Basic stitches used in knitting

Stocking stitch

Garter stitch

Ribbing

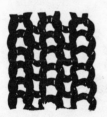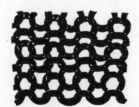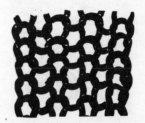

Knit a row, purl a row

Knit all rows

Knitting and purling used together, e.g. K1, P1, K1, P1.

Left-handed knitting

Casting on

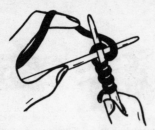 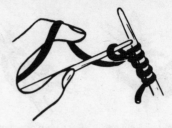

Make a slip knot on the right-hand pin, put left-hand pin in the knot, bring yarn over left-hand pin. When started put left-hand pin between stitches.

Pull the loop made through the stitches and put on right-hand pin.

Knit stitch

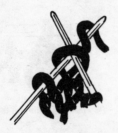 

Put left-hand pin under the stitch on the right-hand pin. Take yarn over left-hand pin.

Pull the loop made through the stitch and slip onto left-hand pin. Slide the bottom part of the stitch off the right-hand pin.

Purl stitch

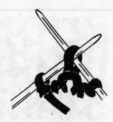

Pass the left-hand pin through the front of the next stitch.

Wrap the yarn around the left-hand pin and bring the yarn and pin backwards to form the new stitch.

Casting off

 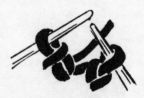

Knit two stitches, using the right-hand pin, slip the first stitch over the second stitch.

Knit the next stitch and continue in the same way.

72

One-handed knitting aids

Gordon knitting aid

This aid from Homecraft Supplies fits easily onto the edge of a table or chair arm and can be used to hold thick or thin knitting pins.

Place the aid in a convenient position at the edge of a table and slide the clamp towards the narrow end until the aid is secure. Open the cylinder by twisting it at the top and insert the knitting pin in between the top or bottom space depending upon the thickness of the pin. (Add a rubber thimble onto the end of the pin before inserting it.) Twist the cylinder at the top until it is secure.

The knitting pin is removed at the end of each row and the other one inserted.

Home-made knitting aid

This is made from a piece of wood cut across the middle at an angle and a wooden base. The grooves can be chiselled or drilled to hold two different sizes of knitting pin, e.g. 10mm and 3mm wide.

A screw to hold the wing nut is inserted into the aid before it is glued to the base.

Suggested sizes:

Base: 13mm × 75mm × 230mm

Block: 45mm × 75mm × 50mm

Angle: 30 degrees

The aid is tightened by screwing down the wing nut. It needs to be clamped onto the edge of a table.

Curtain weights can be used to hold down the knitting.

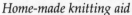

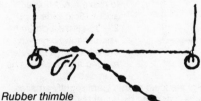

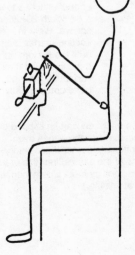

Rubber thimble
Wrap a piece of foam around the end of the knitting pin.

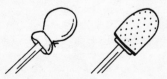

Push on a rubber thimble.

Holding the second knitting pin

The 'working' knitting pin has to be supported by the body while the yarn is wound around the pins. This is picked up when the stitch is being made.

'Easy-to-do' knitting patterns

Using nytrim:

Bag

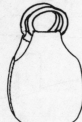

Using 5mm–8mm knitting pins cast on 26 stitches and knit 2 rows. Increase 1 stitch at each end of the next and every alternate row until there are 44 stitches.

Knit 82 rows and then decrease at each end of the next and every alternate row until there are 26 stitches. Knit 2 rows. Cast off.

Stitch up each side of the bag using a bodkin and a piece of the nytrim, fastening each end securely.

Fold each of the top edges through a bag handle and stitch down on the inside with the nytrim. (This bag can be used as a shopping bag or for carrying items in the centre.)

Coat-hanger

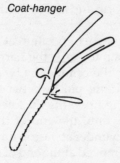

Cast on 6–10 stitches using 5mm–7mm knitting pins. (The knitting has to cover both sides of the coat-hanger and also be overstitched). Knit enough rows to cover the length of the coat-hanger. (If using nytrim, this may stretch so that the length can be shorter.)

Cast off leaving sufficient nytrim to overstitch the edges around the coathanger, e.g. 38–45mm.

Add a ribbon or scented sachet around the hook if it is to be sold.

(These can also be made for use in the centre.)

Using dishcloth cotton:

Dishcloth

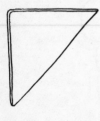

Using 3mm–7mm knitting pins, cast on enough stitches to make a dishcloth 20–25cm square. Work in plain knitting (garter stitch) until the bottom right-hand corner of the cloth can touch the top left-hand corner neatly. Cast off.

The first stitch on each row can be slipped onto the right knitting pin to make the edges even.

Crochet a loop onto one corner if necessary. (Dishcloths are one of the easiest items to make and can usually be done by most elderly people who have some ability at knitting.)

Pot-holder

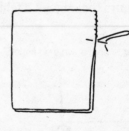

This is made in the same way as the dishcloth except that it is longer so that it can be folded over. Cast on enough stitches to make a pot-holder about 15cm wide e.g. 25–35 stitches on 3mm–7mm knitting pins. Knit the work until it is twice as long as the width and then cast off.

A piece of wadding or thin foam slightly smaller than the pot-holder can be put in between the layers before stitching. Over-stitch the edges. Add a crocheted loop if necessary.

(These items can be trimmed and put in special wrapping for a sale of work.)

French knitting
The yarn is wrapped around pins or nails to give the same effect as knitting.

Using a bobbin

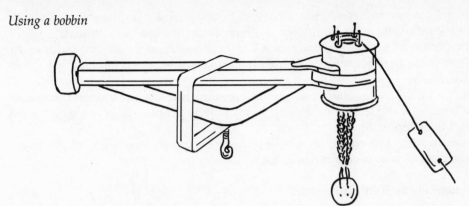

A bobbin may be held by hand or in a Zyliss holder which is clamped onto the corner of a table. The 'wheel' at the end of the holder is turned until the bobbin is secure but can be moved slightly so that the knitting can be done. When the knitting is long enough a curtain weight can be fastened onto it so that the work is held taut. A 'cleat' or weight may be threaded onto the yarn to prevent it from loosening around the pins.

Working the knitting
Using an empty wooden bobbin with four rustproof nails attached at the top or a French knitting bobbin, fasten the end of the yarn loosely over one of the nails. Wrap the yarn over the next nail from the back to the front and proceed until all the nails plus first one are covered. Using an awl or similar tool, lift the lower loop over the upper loop and nail to the back. Wrap the yarn around the second nail and repeat.

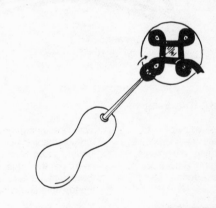

Using a frame

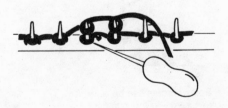

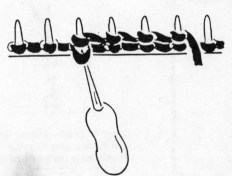

This is worked in the same way as the bobbin except that the frame can be clamped to a table or used over the knees (Romsey knitting frame). Frame knitting can be used to make scarves and other larger items.

A clamp can be used to attach the frame to the table.

LEATHERWORK

Leatherwork can be another creative activity, either for people who just want to thong a kit or for the more able who would like to attempt something a little more difficult.

For the person who enjoys making up a kit, these are usually easy and quick to do although they can be expensive. Using a leather skin is sometimes cheaper, but it has to be cut accurately.

The scope for the craft is enormous, from simple link belt kits and thonged purses to intricate handbags and leather modelling. Many elderly people would probably prefer to attempt the simpler items.

To make up kits, press-stud tools may be the only equipment needed, while the more complicated work may need a range of tools.

Some fastenings used in leatherwork

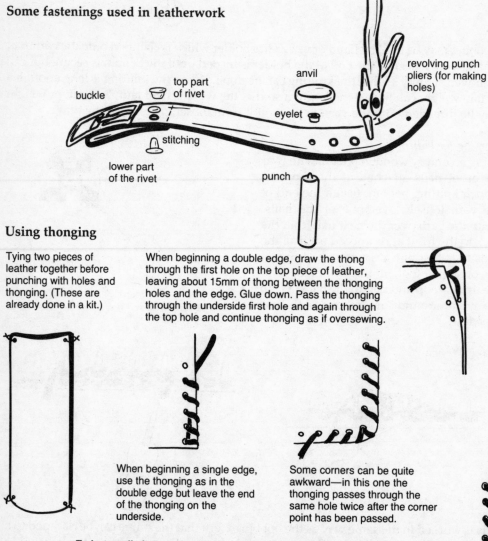

buckle

top part of rivet

anvil

eyelet

revolving punch pliers (for making holes)

stitching

lower part of the rivet

punch

Using thonging

Tying two pieces of leather together before punching with holes and thonging. (These are already done in a kit.)

When beginning a double edge, draw the thong through the first hole on the top piece of leather, leaving about 15mm of thong between the thonging holes and the edge. Glue down. Pass the thonging through the underside first hole and again through the top hole and continue thonging as if oversewing.

When beginning a single edge, use the thonging as in the double edge but leave the end of the thonging on the underside.

Some corners can be quite awkward—in this one the thonging passes through the same hole twice after the corner point has been passed.

To fasten off after passing the thong through the last hole, thread it in between the two leathers under the last hole. Cut off the surplus thong leaving 20mm—glue on the inside.

Making up a belt kit

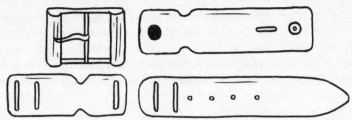

Sample set of pieces in a belt kit

In some belt kits there is only one set of holes for the new link to pass through. In this kit there are more holes, so that the belt is thicker and stronger, but elderly people may find the simpler kit easier to use.

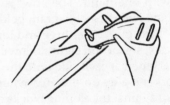

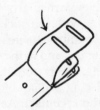

1 Pass the first link through the first hole in the tongue.

2 Pass the next link through three holes.

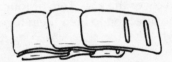

3 Continue passing the links through three holes until the belt is long enough for the user.

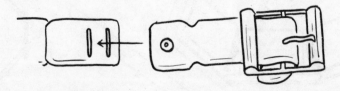

4 Fit the buckle piece onto the buckle and pass through the last set of three holes in the links. Fasten the press-stud.

WORK WITH LOLLIPOP STICKS, MATCHES AND CLOTHES-PEGS

Elderly people enjoy creative activities, but they may not want anything too expensive. In this case, work with lollipop sticks, matches or clothes-pegs may be the answer. They are fairly easy and cheap to obtain, need no tools, and offer scope for quite ambitious projects by those who have a flair for model-making. This kind of activity generally appeals to men, and it can also be done by someone who has the use of only one hand.

Lollipop sticks

Many items can be made from these. Two are given here, but you can find many more ideas, with illustrated instructions, in booklets and leaflets. Both the ideas here use jigs. These are not essential, but elderly people generally find that they make the work easier and give a better result. The size of the jig will depend on the length of sticks chosen, and once decided the jigs can be made out of wood by a local handyman.

A fruitbowl

A good length of stick for this is 11.5cm and the work will be easier if the jig is mounted on a turntable, particularly for someone working with one hand. The bowl is made upside down, with the sticks being placed in alternate layers (see diagram below). It may help to number the jigs first. In the first layer, sticks one, two, three and four are used in sequence, and in the second layer sticks five, six, seven and eight, following the slant of the jig. Apart from the first layer, each stick is glued at each side onto the sticks below by placing a small blob of Evostick woodworker's glue on the area where the sticks have direct contact. As the sticks should lean up against the sloping blocks on the jig, the glue should be placed on the inner edge of the sticks below, a little distance from the edge. When completed the sticks should form a straight line upwards; any sticks that are warped, crooked or damaged should be discarded.

Towards the top (i.e. the bottom of the finished bowl), gradually work inwards by covering only two-thirds of the width of the stick on the previous row. When the gap between the sticks is about 10cm, make the base by first placing a set of sticks side by side on a table until the correct width is achieved to cover the gap. Two or four more sticks are then glued across the sticks in the opposite direction to hold them together. When dry, the base can be glued on to the fruitbowl.

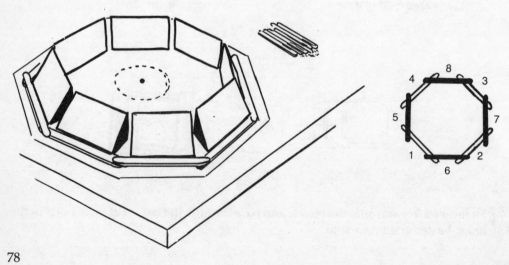

A chalet

Using sticks 14cm long, place them in the jig as shown using two sticks on each layer, a left and a right stick in one direction and a left and right stick in the other direction. Place the glue on the stick underneath where there is direct contact, using sufficient to hold the sticks together without showing on the outside. Glue each stick in sequence until you reach the top of the jig.

The roof is made in the same way, using a jig with triangular pieces of wood. The sticks are placed to slant against the jig pieces and the last stick should complete the covering of the roof. When it is finished a small piece of thin dowelling can be glued in the centre to form a chimney.

Form the base in the same way as for the fruitbowl and glue to the base of the chalet. To finish the chalet, glue 2.5cm mirror tiles to the sides for windows, and stick the ends of two lollipop sticks side by side to form the door. The chalet can also be sprinkled with green shunkle or artificial ferns can be added. Uhu glue is suitable for these trimmings. The inside of the base of the chalet can be lined with foam 3mm thick.

A trinket box can be made in the same way, making a flat lid rather than a sloping roof and gluing small pieces of leather to the inside to form hinges.

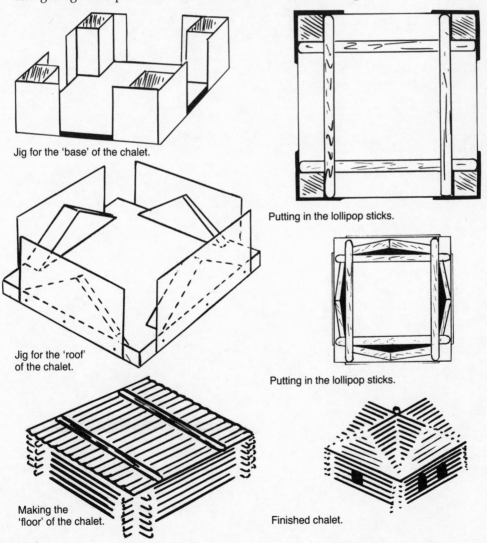

Jig for the 'base' of the chalet.

Putting in the lollipop sticks.

Jig for the 'roof' of the chalet.

Putting in the lollipop sticks.

Making the 'floor' of the chalet.

Finished chalet.

Matchsticks

Matchstick kits can be bought, or you can use ordinary spent matches by cutting off the heads with clippers. Those who are more ambitious can attempt model buildings made out of matchsticks and it is possible to create intricate works of art.

Clothes-pegs

Spring-type clothes-pegs can be used (with the metal clip removed), and many items can be made using Evostick woodworker's glue, including furniture for dolls' houses. It is also possible to buy peg doll kits to make up.

PATCHWORK

This is an activity which can be attempted without a lot of difficulty and expense as odd pieces of material from other activities can be used. A wide range of articles can be made, from tea cosies to bedspreads, and it may be possible to get some of the elderly people to sit together as a group to do some of the larger projects. Templates of the different shapes can be purchased at a local shop or they can be made by hand from card or other strong material. Complete kits can also be bought.

Using a template, mark out the shapes onto a piece of fabric and leave about 7mm of material around each shape to turn underneath. Cut out the shape with the extra material. Mark out the same shapes onto a piece of fairly stiff paper (without the allowance), cut out and place the paper piece onto the wrong side of the fabric shape and pin if necessary. Fold the fabric gently over the paper, following one edge at a time, and tack each side when complete. Press the edges with an iron and lay the completed shapes into a pattern. Oversew the edges together, remove the paper and tacking threads and press again. Add additional material underneath the shapes or around the edges if necessary.

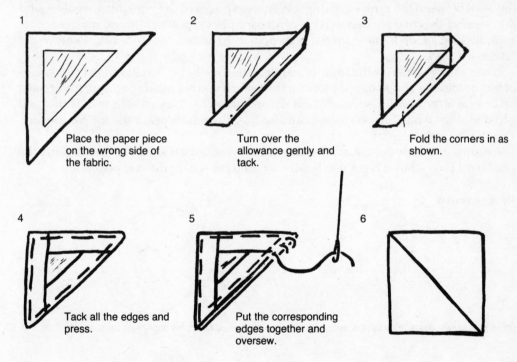

1 Place the paper piece on the wrong side of the fabric.

2 Turn over the allowance gently and tack.

3 Fold the corners in as shown.

4 Tack all the edges and press.

5 Put the corresponding edges together and oversew.

6

POM-POM TOYS

Sometimes it may be very difficult to find an activity that an elderly person can manage to do. He may have limited mental faculties, or be so disabled that most activities are impossible or unsafe for him.

People like this may be able to make a simple pom-pom toy—two woollen balls knotted together to make the head and body of, say, an Easter chicken. These toys are easy to make, need no tools or equipment and can be done by someone in bed or with a severe visual impairment. All you will need are a few pairs of cardboard rings, several small balls of wool, some oddments of felt and glue.

To make a pom-pom toy, cut two pairs of cardboard rings, one pair slightly smaller than the other. They can be any size, but useful sizes are small rings 10cm across with a 4cm hole and larger rings 13.5cm across with a 4.5cm hole. Using 4-ply or 6-ply wool in an appropriate colour (yellow for a chicken), wind several small balls of wool which will pass through the holes in the centre of the rings. Take one pair of rings and start to wrap the wool round both pieces, showing the elderly person how it is done. When the pair of rings is fully wrapped and the centre hole is nearly full, take a pair of scissors and cut the wool between the cardboard rings. Wrap two pieces of the remaining wool around the centre of the cut wool between the cardboard pieces, pull tightly and make a secure knot, leaving a loop to hang up the pom-pom or to tie onto another ball. Remove the cardboard pieces.

When the two balls for the toy are complete, tie together securely and cut two circles of felt for the eyes and a shaped piece for the beak. If you are making an animal such as a cat or a rabbit, you will also need to cut shaped pieces for the ears. These are fitted and glued into the wool. Shaped pieces can also be glued underneath the toy for the feet. Trim with a ribbon around the neck.

A confused elderly person may be able to do no more than wrap the wool around the cardboard pieces but can get much satisfaction from seeing the completed toy.

Items needed

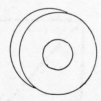

Small pair of cardboard rings for the head.

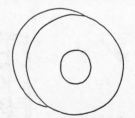

Larger pair of cardboard rings for the body.

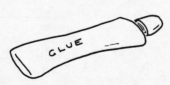

Glue to stick felt pieces into the wool.

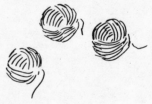

Small balls of wool.

Kits
Pom-pom toy kits are available in some toy shops.

Making a pom-pom toy

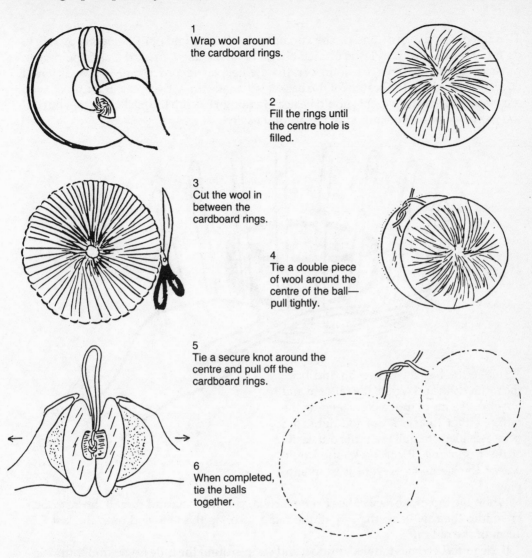

1
Wrap wool around the cardboard rings.

2
Fill the rings until the centre hole is filled.

3
Cut the wool in between the cardboard rings.

4
Tie a double piece of wool around the centre of the ball—pull tightly.

5
Tie a secure knot around the centre and pull off the cardboard rings.

6
When completed, tie the balls together.

Felt pieces for the toy—these can usually be stuck on with Uhu glue.

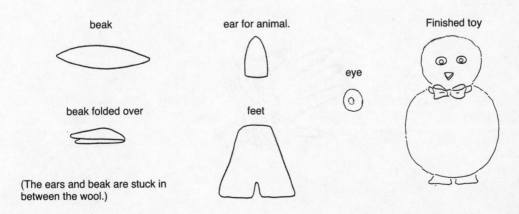

beak

beak folded over

(The ears and beak are stuck in between the wool.)

ear for animal.

feet

eye

Finished toy

RAFFIA WORK

This activity is easy to do and can be attempted with one hand or by someone unable to do more difficult work. Plastic or metal baskets can be used, or cards, and the person can use different textures or colours of raffia, twine, plastic cord or cane to give different effects. A weight in the bottom of the basket will make the activity easier for those who are one-handed. The weight should be heavy enough to keep the basket secure, but not too heavy—the basket should move around easily.

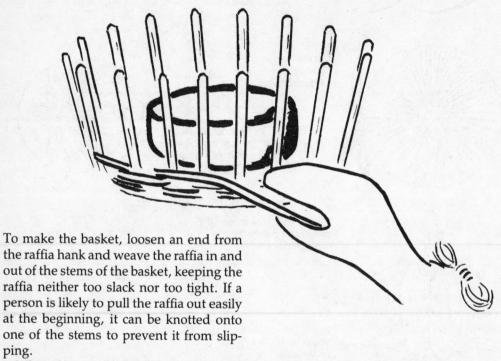

To make the basket, loosen an end from the raffia hank and weave the raffia in and out of the stems of the basket, keeping the raffia neither too slack nor too tight. If a person is likely to pull the raffia out easily at the beginning, it can be knotted onto one of the stems to prevent it from slipping.

When the top of the basket has been reached, cut the raffia and thread the last 7.5cm or so into the row beneath. To join the raffia, overlap the new end onto the last 7.5–10cm of the old raffia.

If the raffia becomes tangled, undo it and wrap around the little finger and thumb in a figure of eight, wrapping the last few centimetres round the middle of the bundle in half-hitches.

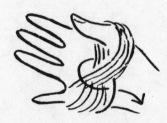

RUG-MAKING

This useful craft, popular with both men and women, can be done in several ways. Rugs can be stitched, using long lengths of rug wool and a bodkin to sew stitches such as double cross-stitch, or they can be pegged, using a rug hook with short lengths of rug wool. The canvas can be bought in different widths off a roll or it may be part of a kit, with a pattern marked on it. Even those who have a visual impairment can make rugs, but they may need a sighted person to peg the outline of the pattern before they begin.

Rug-making may be done with two hands or one-handed, by attaching the canvas to a home-made frame which can be clamped onto a table or chair arm. If two people are working on a pegged rug at the same time from opposite directions, one will need to use the one-handed method while the other works with both hands, so that the pile of the wool lies in the same direction. If they are working from the same end they must follow the same method.

Some elderly people who are frail or have a serious heart condition may find this activity a little strenuous, and someone with a chest complaint may have difficulty in working with certain types of wool.

It may be best for a person to start with a small plain rug before attempting a larger or more ambitious one, but once he has become proficient he may like to experiment with his own designs and colours.

NOTE: If the rug wool is thin, several strands may have to be worked together.

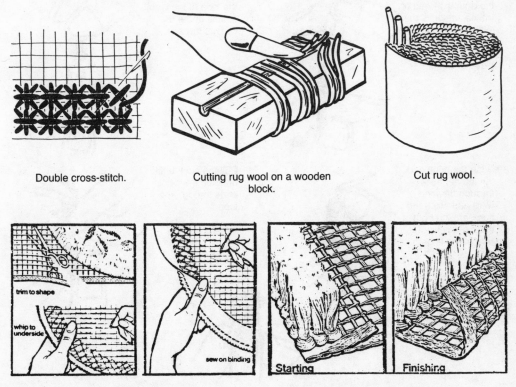

Double cross-stitch.

Cutting rug wool on a wooden block.

Cut rug wool.

Finishing off a circular or stitched rug.

Starting and finishing a 'pegged' rug.

Rug-making techniques

One-handed method

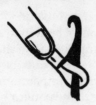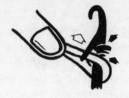

1   Place a piece of folded, cut wool behind the latchet.

2   Push the hook down through one square and up through the one immediately in front.

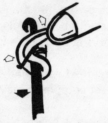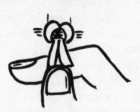

3   Put the two ends of the wool into the 'eye' of the hook and pull the hook back through the loop, giving it a flick upwards at the same time.

4   Pull lightly on the two ends of the wool to tighten the knot.

Two-handed method

1   Push the hook under the double thread of the canvas until the latchet is through the canvas, then catch the loop of a folded piece of wool.

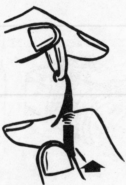

2   Pull the hook until the loop of the wool comes under the canvas threads.

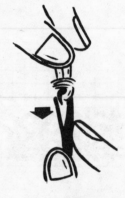

3   Push the hook and the latchet back through the loop of wool and catch the hook around both ends of the wool held in the fingers.

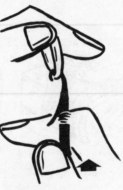

4   Pull the hook back, bringing the wool ends through the loop.

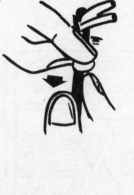

5   Pull lightly on the two ends of wool to tighten the knot.

SEWING

This is a popular activity which elderly people may be able to do without too much difficulty. Some may enjoy simple hand-sewing, such as making draught-excluders, aprons and cushions, while others may prefer more intricate work.

Simple patterns (for example, McCall's easy stitch patterns) are available for anyone who would like to try dressmaking. If a person has a deformity, the pattern may need to be altered to fit.

In hand-sewing, a person with the use of only one hand may like to try using a foam wedge covered in vinyl. Non-slip material is stitched on top of the wedge to prevent the material from slipping, and also underneath to stop the wedge from slipping off the table.

To help those with a disability there are self-threading needles, pincushions which clip onto the wrist, left-handed scissors and easy-to-use scissors, pendant magnifiers which hang around the neck and magnifiers that clamp onto a table or chair arm, needle threaders, pins with large heads, and Helping Hands, special pick-up sticks with magnets for retrieving pins and so on.

Foam wedge for a one-handed sewer

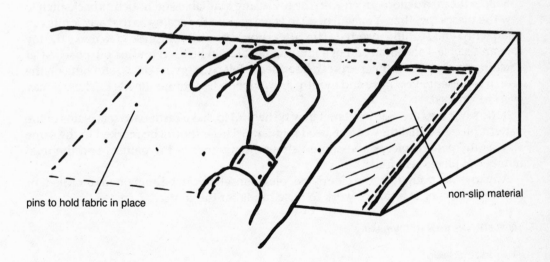

pins to hold fabric in place

non-slip material

Self-threading needle

Needles may be inserted into a firm surface (e.g. cork or a pin cushion) for threading with one hand.

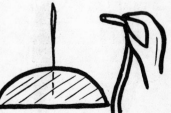

SOFT TOYS

Some elderly people enjoy making soft toys, particularly if they have grandchildren or other young relatives. Simple toy kits are usually easy to make, although the elderly person needs to be able to see, use a needle and thread safely and understand any instructions. Toy kits are often expensive, so if one or more people enjoy making them it may be worthwhile buying a length of fur fabric or similar material, a bag of stuffing and the eyes, felt, cottons, ribbon and joints separately. Pliers may be needed to attach the eyes and fix any joints.

When using a length of fur fabric, place it on a table face downwards so that the pattern pieces can be marked out on the back—be sure to check the direction of the pile, nap or design before doing this. Some pattern pieces are paired—that is, each body part, such as the arms and legs, has two pieces—and when cutting these out the pattern piece should be reversed the second time so that the two pieces can be sewn together in the same direction. It is wise to check that there is enough material before cutting out the pieces.

After the pieces have been cut out, add any safety eyes to the head pieces (these may have a stem and fastener or a stalk which has to be twisted and compressed with pliers); the ears can be added after the head pieces have been sewn together. Ears can be strengthened with buckram or similar stiff material, or lightly padded.

Follow the instructions given with the toy, using a suitable stitch such as backstitch to sew the pieces together. You will need to leave gaps in the seams so that any joints can be attached and stuffing inserted. The latter should be well compressed to make the toy firm and stable—the knob end of a knitting needle can be used for this purpose. After stitching up the gaps, other parts can be added—felt pads on the paws, stitching on the face to represent eyes, nose and mouth, and a ribbon tied round the neck. The toy may even be dressed.

If the same toys are made often, it may be helpful to make cardboard templates of the pattern pieces so that they can be used regularly. These should be marked in the same way as the pattern pieces and should show the number of the pattern and the total number of pieces required.

Any toys not bought by the elderly people themselves can be auctioned or raffled, or sold to visitors or at a sale of work to raise funds for the centre.

Some stitches used in toymaking

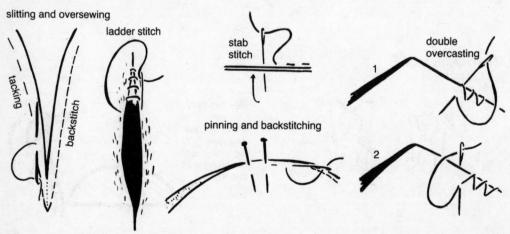

Making a soft toy

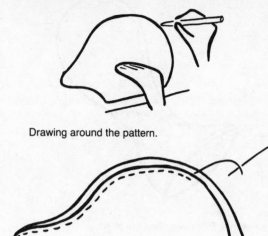

Drawing around the pattern.

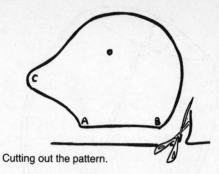

Cutting out the pattern.

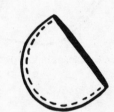

head (two pieces)

Stitching in the head gusset.

The ear has four pieces.

The ear may be sewn into the seam or added afterwards.

Attaching safety eyes

After putting the stem of the eye through a hole in the material, press on the disc. This is usually done by hand, but sometimes a tool may be needed. (The teeth of the disc should face away from the eye.) When complete, check that the eye is secure.

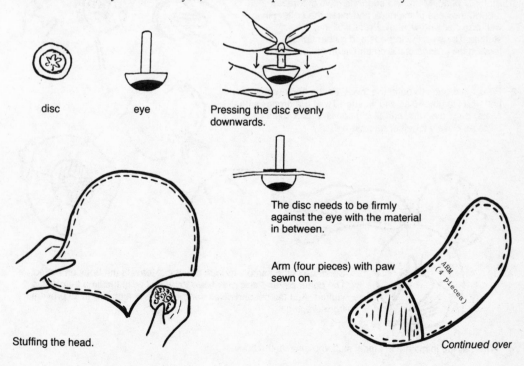

disc

eye

Pressing the disc evenly downwards.

The disc needs to be firmly against the eye with the material in between.

Arm (four pieces) with paw sewn on.

ARM (4 pieces)

Stuffing the head.

Continued over

Body   Leg

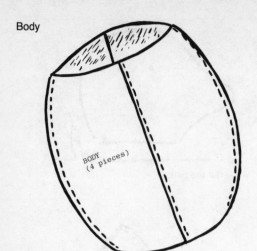

This may be two pieces or four pieces.   The leg has four pieces and two soles.

Adding the joints

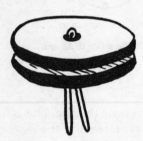

Cotter pin and discs (and washers).

Cross-section of a 'joint'   stuffing

1   Stuff the head. Make two separate rows of threads around the base of the neck and insert the cotter pin with one disc and washer. Press well into the stuffing. Draw up the threads and gather tightly, leaving the prongs of the cotter pin on the outside.

2   Pass the prongs through the 'neck' on the body (unstuffed) and add the other disc and washer. Twist the prongs with pliers, bend over and curl at the edges, pushing the two discs as closely together as possible.

3

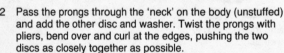

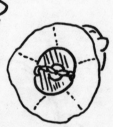

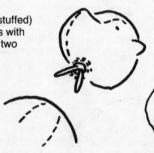

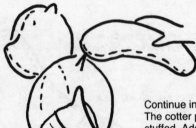

Continue in the same way with the limbs, leaving the body unstuffed. The cotter pin and disc may have to be placed in the limb before it is stuffed. Add the second disc over the first one temporarily to prevent it from slipping.

4   When all the joints are in place, stuff and sew up the body.

7 GAMES

BINGO

This light-hearted game can give elderly people much fun and pleasure, particularly if there are prizes to be won.

Each person has a bingo card with 15 numbers which he has to cover as they are called out. The first person to fill his card shouts, 'Bingo!' and wins the game. The numbers can be covered with normal counters, small squares of wood, painted ridged bottle tops, or they may be specially adapted so that people with poor hand function can hold them more easily. If someone is partially sighted, it may be possible to blow up the bingo card on a photocopying machine, or to mark out a card with larger numbers. The new card can then be stuck down on a stronger piece of card and covered with transparent Fablon to make it more hardwearing. Blind players may like to use a plastic bingo board with shutters which can be adapted with braille markings. These can be put on Tenza tape and stuck beside each number on the board. The braille numbers are made by using a braille frame and awl, obtainable from the RNIB. Ideally, a blind

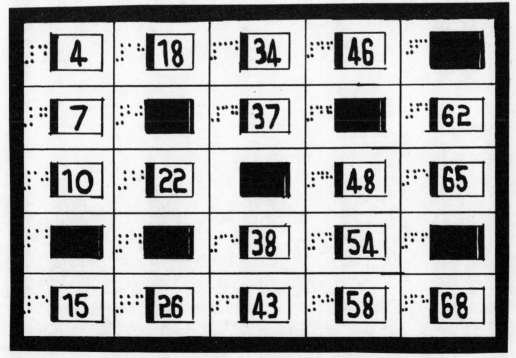

Adapted bingo board for the blind (it may be possible to get rejects from amusement arcades).
Bingo 'shutter trays' are also available from Winslow Press. They also supply large print Bingo cards.

person should have his own bingo board so that he can memorise the numbers beforehand.

The caller has a bag of numbered discs, and as she calls each number she places it on a marked board. When a person shouts 'Bingo!' his card can be checked against the board.

To make the game more fun, certain names can be used with some of the numbers. These incude:

Kelly's eye—No. 1

Downing Street—No. 10

Legs eleven—No. 11

Coming of age—18

Key of the door—21

Two little ducks—22

Clickety-click—66

Two fat ladies—88

Top of the house—90

and so on.

On its own—No. 1, 2, etc.

Blind 20, 30, etc.

All the twos, threes

Those who are deaf may find it easier to play if they can sit near the front and face the caller.

To play, the participants may pay for each game or a number of games and the money raised can be used to buy prizes. Large bags of miniature sweets such as Mars bars have been found to be popular prizes and they are inexpensive to buy. Care needs to be taken to see that the prize is suitable for the person receiving it—for example, a person with diabetes will need diabetic sweets or a different prize.

BILLIARDS AND SNOOKER

These can be popular games in a centre, particularly if there are people who enjoy watching or playing them. They are not too strenuous for elderly people and can be used in competitions either in the centre or between centres. Players with the use of only one hand may be able to rest the cue over the wrist of the affected hand, or it can be placed through the bristles of an upturned brush. An aid can also be bought to support the cue. People in wheelchairs usually need a shorter cue and may require assistance from the staff from time to time.

Billiards

This is a more intricate game than snooker and may be less popular with some elderly people who may have difficulty in remembering the various rules. The aim of the game is to score as many points as possible and to reach a certain number of points or lead after a certain length of time. Points can be scored by hitting the other two balls in the same shot or by potting a ball. This may be the cue ball which has hit another ball, or it may be the other ball itself.

Snooker

In snooker the object of the game is to pot the coloured balls into the pockets around the table. This has to be done in sequence—a red ball, then a coloured ball, and so on until all the red balls are off the table. (The coloured balls are retrieved and replaced on their 'spot'.) When only the coloured balls remain, these have to be potted in order according to their number of points—yellow (two points), green (three points), brown (four points), blue (five points), pink (six points) and black (seven points). The red balls count as one point each. The person with the higher number of points wins the game.

Equipment needed for both games is quite simple—a cue for each player, chalk (to roughen the end of the cue), three balls for billiards (one red and two white), 22 balls for snooker (one white, 15 red and one of each of the six colours), a triangle to position the red balls, a scoring board and a billiards/snooker table. A full-sized table is 12 feet long, but a smaller table may be more suitable for a centre; others have folding legs, or a table top can be placed on top of a normal table (this may need to be clamped to make it secure).

Two ways of supporting a cue using one hand

A person who has had a stroke may be able to control a cue on top of the wrist on the affected side.

Non-slip material under a flat brush may help to prevent it from slipping.

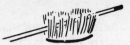

Setting up a table for billiards or snooker

Billards

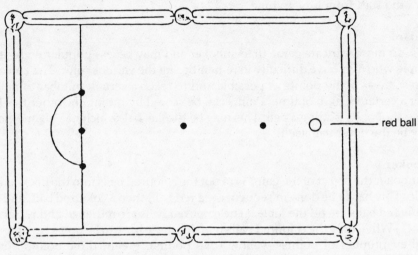

— red ball

Balls: ○ White ball   } given to each of
       ⊙ White ball with spots } the players
       ○ Red ball placed on 'The Spot'

Snooker

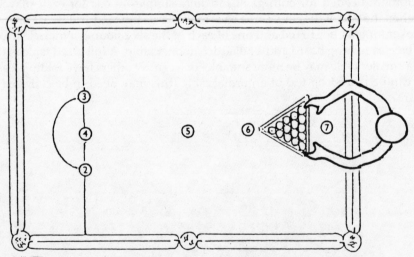

Balls: ○ White 'cue-ball' is placed in the 'D'   ⑤ Blue ball on the 'centre spot'
       ② Yellow ball } these are placed on   ⑥ Pink ball on the 'pyramid spot'
       ③ Green ball } the 'baulk line'   ⑦ Black ball on 'the spot'
       ④ Brown ball }

The fifteen red balls are placed in the triangle which is then removed. The space in the 'D' is used to start the game with a white ball or if a coloured ball has been pocketed and has to be returned to the table.

CHESS

Chess is a more complicated game, but it can be a useful activity in a centre where the elderly people have normal mental abilities. It can be adapted by using magnetic chessmen and boards, or the RNIB supply several different kinds of chess game for people with poor hand control, tremor or visual handicap. These include sets with pegged pieces that fit into holes in the board. Chessmen can be bought in different shapes and sizes to suit the players. In some centres a computer game may be available, and small travelling chess sets can also be used. A non-slip mat or material placed under the board will prevent it from slipping.

Sometimes staff may be able to organise chess matches between players in the same centre or from other centres, and to award a trophy or other prize to the winner.

Since chess is quite an intricate game, it would be a good idea for staff to study a book on the subject and perhaps have a practice first before offering it to the elderly people!

Pieces on a chess board

On the top row from left to right:

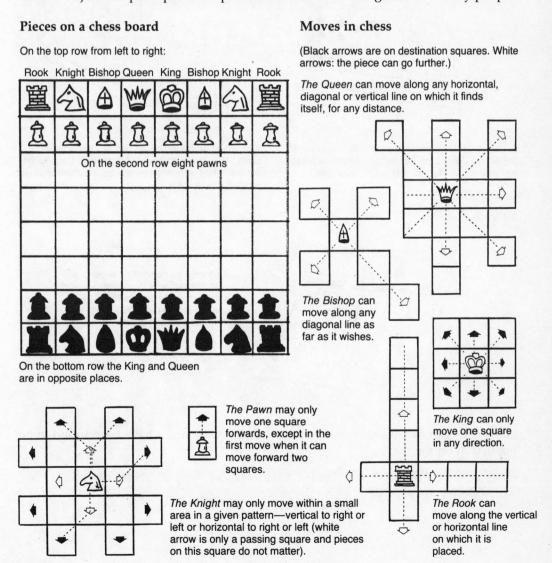

Rook Knight Bishop Queen King Bishop Knight Rook

On the second row eight pawns

On the bottom row the King and Queen are in opposite places.

Moves in chess

(Black arrows are on destination squares. White arrows: the piece can go further.)

The Queen can move along any horizontal, diagonal or vertical line on which it finds itself, for any distance.

The Bishop can move along any diagonal line as far as it wishes.

The King can only move one square in any direction.

The Rook can move along the vertical or horizontal line on which it is placed.

The Pawn may only move one square forwards, except in the first move when it can move forward two squares.

The Knight may only move within a small area in a given pattern—vertical to right or left or horizontal to right or left (white arrow is only a passing square and pieces on this square do not matter).

CARD GAMES

Some elderly people enjoy playing card games and these can be an entertaining pastime in a centre. People usually know which games they want to play, have similar abilities and can organise themselves into a group, but sometimes this may not be so, and then staff will need to help to arrange a group, suggest games or provide aids or assistance.

Aids are available which will hold cards if a person is 'one-handed' or has difficulty in controlling them and some cards are adapted for people who are visually impaired, with braille or moon markings or larger symbols.

Card holders

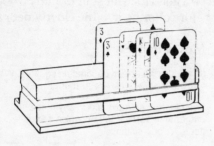

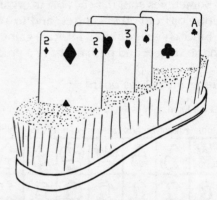

A wooden card holder with an elastic band around the centre can be used to support cards. (A plastic one without an elastic band is also available.)

An unused, upturned brush can be used to hold cards. This needs to have a flat base so that it does not 'rock' Non-slip material can be put underneath to prevent it from slipping.

Patience Board

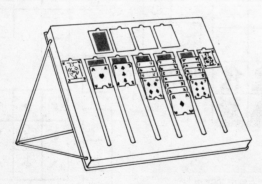

This may be needed by someone who has difficulty in controlling cards when playing Patience. It can be used either while lying down or sitting at a table.

Many card games are available, but the following two games have been found to be popular in centres:

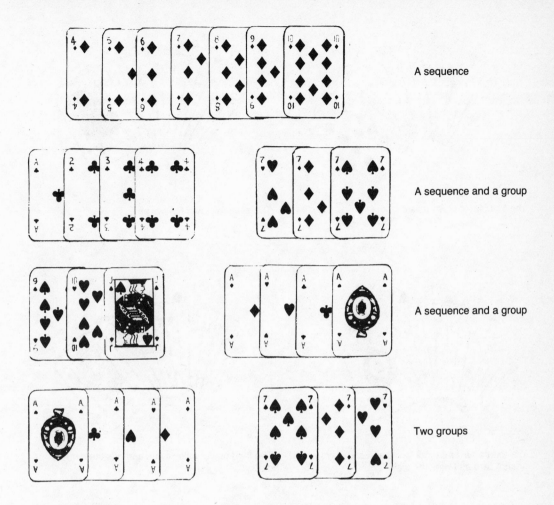

A sequence

A sequence and a group

A sequence and a group

Two groups

This game can be played by two to six players and the aim is to get a 'sequence' or a 'group' (a sequence is three or more cards which follow on in the same suit; a group is three or four cards of the same value from different suits).

After shuffling the cards, they are dealt to each person: ten cards each for two players, seven cards each for three to four players and six cards each for five or six players. The remaining cards are put into a 'stockpile' face downwards in the centre of the table, the top card is put face upwards alongside in the 'discard pile'.

Each player arranges the cards in his hand into sequences or groups. When it is his turn, he takes a card from either the discard pile or the stockpile and returns a card to the discard pile which he does not want.

The first person to get a sequence, a sequence and a group or two groups wins the game. In a centre it may be easier to add up the number of winning games rather than score points.

NOTE: An ace can be '1' or it can follow the King.

Whist

1

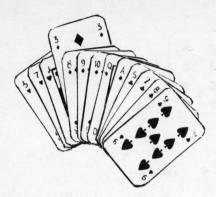

The first player plays a card.

2

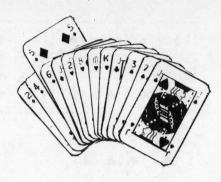

The second player follows suit.

4

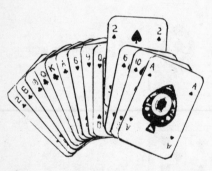

The fourth player cannot follow suit and plays a 'trump' card and wins the trick.

3

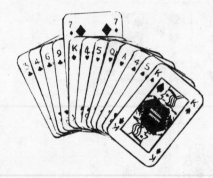

The third player follows suit and has the highest card.

Whist is a game for four players. The aim is to get as many 'tricks' as possible (a trick is the four cards in the centre of the table).

To begin, the dealer 'cuts' the pack and the next card is the 'trump' card (a card of the same suit can beat other cards).

The dealer deals out all the cards (except the jokers) to the players who then arrange them in suits. The player on the left of the dealer starts the game and plays a card (any card) and the other players 'follow suit' (that is, play a card from the same suit). The person with the highest card wins the trick and this is put in a pile beside him. He then plays a card to start the next trick.

If a player does not have a card of the same suit, he may play another card or a trump card and win the trick. If two players play trump cards, the one with the highest card wins the trick.

Play continues until all the cards have been played. The player (or pair of players) with the most tricks wins the game.

To start again, the dealer shuffles the cards and cuts them to find the new trump card for the next game.

98

Patience

Patience games can be played by someone who is unable to play card games with anyone else. These may be quite simple or very complicated.

If a person has difficulty in laying out cards on a table or could disturb them, he may be able to use a patience board.

Here are some games that are easy to play:

Memory game

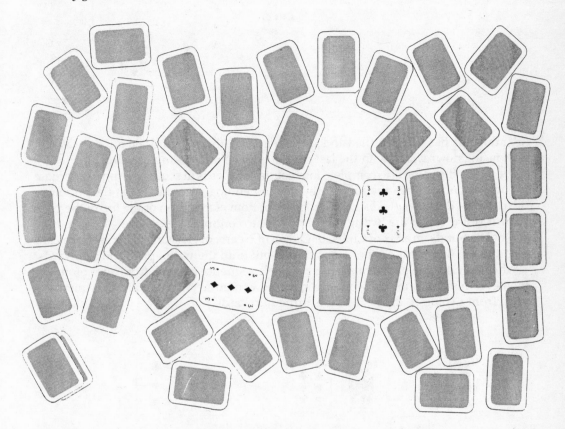

After the pack has been shuffled, the cards are placed face downwards on a table at random. The aim of the game is for the player to try and remember where all the cards are and 'pair' them off.

At each turn, he places two cards face upwards; if these 'match'—have the same value, for example two Kings, two Sevens—they are removed from the table. If not he returns them to their place again, face downwards.

He continues with the game until all the cards have been paired off.

If there is more than one player, the person with the most pairs wins the game.

Klondyke

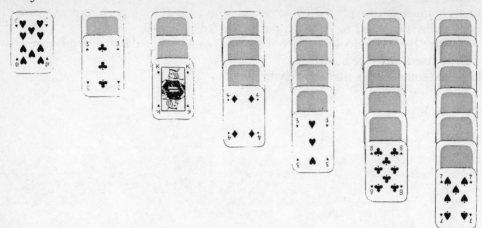

After the pack has been shuffled and jokers removed, the cards are laid out on a table in rows facing downwards with the last card in each column facing upwards.

The aim of the game is to complete four columns of cards in sequence and in alternate colours, beginning with the King at the top and ending with the Ace at the bottom.

To do this, the player takes a card from the bottom of a column or the top of the pack of cards or the top of the 'waste-pile', and tries to continue a sequence—for example, Five of Diamonds on a Six of Clubs, or Queen of Hearts over a King of Spades. If a card from the top of the pack is not wanted, it is put onto the waste-pile facing upwards.

While playing, the person may move a whole sequence of cards from one column to another if this continues the sequence in the new column. (When a card or sequence is taken from a column, the next card is turned upwards.)

Royal Marriage

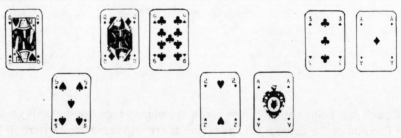

In the game above, the Nine and Three of Clubs can be removed after the Two and Ace of Spades have been taken off the table.

This is an easy game of Patience to play. The aim is to bring the Queen of Hearts and King of Hearts cards together.

After removing the jokers, the player shuffles the cards and places the Queen of Hearts on the table at the left-hand side; the King of Hearts is put at the bottom of the pack. Taking a card from the top of the pack each time, he makes a row of cards starting from the Queen of Hearts. If a card (or pair of cards) has a card on each side of the same suit or value, the card (or cards) in between is removed from the table. The remaining cards are moved together. When the King of Hearts meets the Queen of Hearts, the game is won.

100

GUESSING GAMES

Blockbusters
When playing this game, questions can be chosen to suit the person being asked. Waddingtons make a small version of the game seen on television, and there was also a series of Blockbuster books.

Crosswords
Some elderly people enjoy doing crosswords. Most newspapers publish puzzles of varying difficulty, and whole books of crosswords can be bought from bookshops. These are particularly useful in a centre as they can be used by people sitting in a chair or in bed. Some puzzle magazines are published at monthly intervals and it may be worth placing a regular order for these if someone in the centre enjoys doing them.

Quizzes
These are often popular in a centre, and are a particularly good form of activity where there are plenty of able elderly people. They are easy to organise and can be made more interesting by having teams and keeping scores. Winslow Press produce a quiz book and sets of quiz cards which can be used with elderly people. The questions are graded under different subjects.

Tell me . . .
In this game someone picks a card with a question and a dial is spun to give a letter of the alphabet. When the dial stops the person has to give an answer beginning with the letter shown on the dial. As a substitute, two piles of cards can be used—question cards and alphabet cards. *Tell Me . . .* is made by J. W. Spears.

Trivial pursuit
This can be a challenging game for elderly people who are able enough to take part. Questions need to be suitable for the person who is answering them and it may be helpful to have some simple ones ready in case they are needed. Both normal and children's versions are available, and the latter may be more appropriate for some elderly people.

Many other games are available in addition to the few mentioned here, but these may stimulate ideas.

If a person has poor hand control or other disabilities which prevent him from taking part in an activity, it may be possible to ask someone to help him, perhaps a relative, or else a volunteer or member of staff.

Games are usually available locally from toyshops, sports shops or stationers, but if you cannot obtain them in your area you may have to write to the manufacturers for information (see the Appendices for addresses). Some games are sold separately and boxed, while others are in a compendium. Although these are usually cheaper, the individual ones tend to be sturdier and better for withstanding the wear and tear of use in a centre.

TABLE GAMES

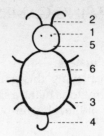

Beetle

In this game, each player has a pencil and paper and throws a dice in turn. Starting with six for the body, a beetle is drawn by adding a piece to the body according to the number thrown on the dice. The first person to complete the beetle wins the game.

A 3D version of Beetle is available from the RNIB for those who have difficulty in seeing a drawing or using a pencil. Beetle cards can also be bought and can be enlarged on a photocopier to make them easier to use.

Dominoes

This popular game is easy to play and organise. Dominoes are made in different forms to suit those who have specific difficulties—for example, coloured dominoes can be used if someone is slightly confused or has a problem in understanding numbers, and those issued by the RNIB are useful for people who have a visual problem. They have raised dots and are easy to see and hold. The RNIB also produce a wooden support for dominoes, for those who are unable to hold the pieces.

Picture dominoes, although intended for children, may be suitable for a confused elderly person who enjoys playing with them. The pictures must be appropriate for an older person.

Draughts

This is another game that elderly people may ask to play. It can be adapted by using a magnetic board and 'men' or a wooden board with sunken squares if a person has a tendency to knock the pieces off the board. The magnetic board, available from Nottingham Rehab, is particularly useful as it can be propped at an angle to suit the people who are playing. The same company also produces a version of the game with interlocking pieces.

Ludo

Some adults still enjoy this game. Different versions are available to suit those who have limited hand control. Nottingham Rehab make a magnetic game and a large-size wooden version with a board 53cm square. It is expensive, but ideal for those who cannot hold normal counters. The RNIB has a ludo game with pegged counters that fit into holes in the board, useful either for those unable to see clearly or for those liable to knock the pieces off the board. Frustration, by M.B. Games, is excellent for elderly people as the counters cannot be dislodged and the dice is 'thrown' by pressing a container in the centre of the board.

Scrabble

This is an interesting game for the more able so long as they have sufficient control to hold the pieces. It can be played with a 'Travel Scrabble' set, which has pieces with legs that fit into holes, or with the RNIB version which has sunken squares to take the tiles. The latter have raised markings for identification. Both these versions would be suitable for people who are likely to knock the pieces. A Giant Scrabble set from Nottingham Rehab has a board 47cm square, with larger letter tiles that are easy to hold.

Scrabble can be played by several people, although one person can play on his own by trying to beat his own score for each game. Non-slip material can be used underneath the board to prevent it from slipping, or it can be put on a turntable.

WORD-FINDING GAMES

These can be popular with the elderly and are also easy to organise. They can be done using a board in front of the group or at a table using a piece of paper.

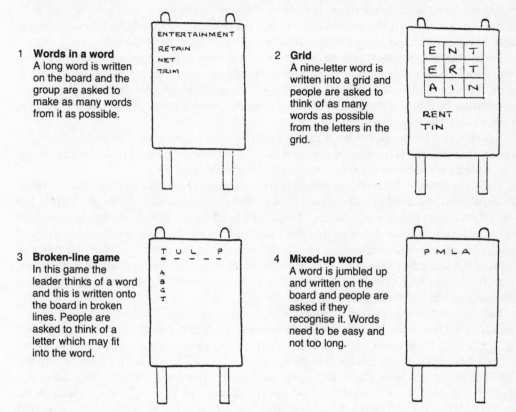

1 **Words in a word**
A long word is written on the board and the group are asked to make as many words from it as possible.

2 **Grid**
A nine-letter word is written into a grid and people are asked to think of as many words as possible from the letters in the grid.

3 **Broken-line game**
In this game the leader thinks of a word and this is written onto the board in broken lines. People are asked to think of a letter which may fit into the word.

4 **Mixed-up word**
A word is jumbled up and written on the board and people are asked if they recognise it. Words need to be easy and not too long.

Equipment

To play some games, it is useful to have a board in front of the group, such as a blackboard, flip-chart or a 'drywipe' board. It should be possible to obtain one of these from a local shop, but if not a supplier may be able to give details (see Appendices for addresses).

To avoid buying a chalkboard, blackboard paint can be used on a piece of wood. Boards can be held by hand or propped against a wall on a table, but it is easier if they can be fixed on a wall or supported on a stand.

JIGSAWS

Some elderly people enjoy making up jigsaw puzzles. These may be quite small—32 pieces—or very large, with perhaps 4,000 pieces or more. Wooden pieces are easier to hold and more suitable for those who have difficulty in holding card pieces, and they are also easier to see if the person has a visual problem. Care should be taken to ensure that any puzzles used have pictures that are suitable for elderly people.

Once a suitable jigsaw has been chosen, you will need to find a jigsaw board or tray—this should be non-slip or have a lip round the edge to prevent any pieces falling off. It must be larger than the jigsaw. If a tray is not available (catering trolley trays can sometimes be used), you may be able to make one from a piece of wood with beading round the edge (see opposite).

Jigsaws can be made up by a person on his own or may be a joint venture and completed by several people, perhaps working at different times. In this case the jigsaw can be left on a table in an area where it will not be disturbed.

Finished jigsaws can be dismantled for future use, or they may be glued onto a piece of hardboard, covered in transparent Fablon and hung on a wall. To do this, cover the completed jigsaw with a piece of thin wood and, holding the wood and tray very firmly, turn the jigsaw upside down so that the picture is facing downwards. Remove the tray and, using a general-purpose glue such as Uhu, cover the entire surface of a piece of hardboard and press the glued side onto the back of the jigsaw. Leave to dry and then turn the jigsaw face upwards again. Cover in transparent Fablon, screw fittings onto the back of the hardboard and hang on a wall.

Fablon needs to be applied with care and the process should not be hurried. Start by securing the hardboard by placing it on a non-slip surface or fixing it to the work surface with Blu-tac. Then open approximately 5–10cm of Fablon and stick about 5cm to the work surface beside the jigsaw. Gently loosen the roll of Fablon, without removing the backing paper, to check that it will cover the jigsaw. Wind the roll and, starting at the right-hand side, allow 1cm or so of Fablon to fall onto the jigsaw. Using a clean cloth, gently rub this up and down the jigsaw from the top edge to the bottom, ensuring that there are no creases in the Fablon. Gradually unwind the Fablon (you may need a second person to do this) and fold up the backing paper as the Fablon is slowly pressed onto the jigsaw. Keep a steady rhythmic movement with the cloth so that no creases form. When the jigsaw is covered, cut the Fablon, leaving about 5cm around the edge to be folded over the hardboard at the back.

You may prefer to experiment on another item before trying it on the jigsaw. You can also frame the jigsaw like a picture.

Attach the wood to the work surface using Blu-tac or non-slip matting.

Backing paper

Stick the edge of the Fablon onto the work surface to secure it.

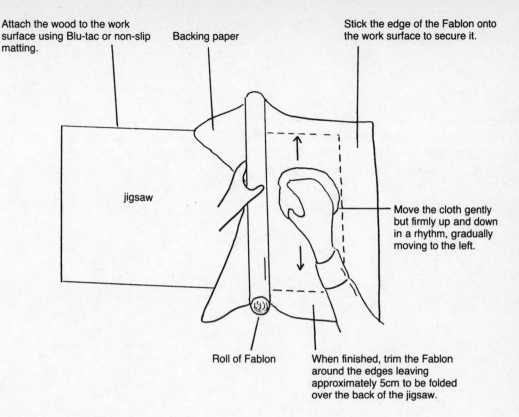

jigsaw

Move the cloth gently but firmly up and down in a rhythm, gradually moving to the left.

Roll of Fablon

When finished, trim the Fablon around the edges leaving approximately 5cm to be folded over the back of the jigsaw.

Making a jigsaw tray

Cut a piece of plywood or hardboard larger than the size of jigsaw to be used.

Useful sizes are:
46 × 30.5cm for
the smaller puzzles

61 × 46cm for
53 × 40cm puzzle

91.5 × 61cm
76 × 53cm puzzle

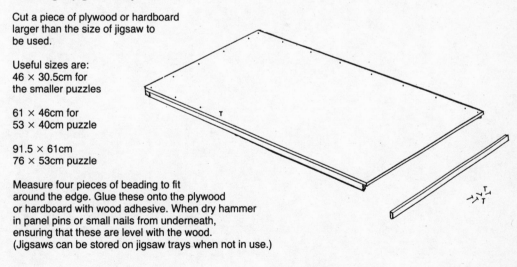

Measure four pieces of beading to fit around the edge. Glue these onto the plywood or hardboard with wood adhesive. When dry hammer in panel pins or small nails from underneath, ensuring that these are level with the wood.
(Jigsaws can be stored on jigsaw trays when not in use.)

Aid

Insert a hat pin or normal pin through a piece of cork.

A person with limited hand function may be able to use this to 'stab' the cardboard pieces.

8 OTHER ACTIVITIES

BAKING

This can be an enjoyable activity for elderly people in a centre. It gives them a sense of purpose, and an opportunity to show their skill and contribute to the running of the centre.

Cakes and buns are popular favourites, although some people may be able to attempt more ambitious ideas. If a group of people want to take part in the activity, it may be possible to split it up so that different people are doing different activities—one person weighing ingredients and others mixing them, and so on. Others may be willing to do the more simple tasks like washing up or laying the table.

If the people are quite fit they may be able to work in a normal kitchen, but others may prefer to sit at a table if a low work surface is not available in the kitchen. In some centres it may be safer and more convenient to keep the elderly people away from the kitchen and to use a table in another room.

Aids are available if anyone needs to use them. These include non-slip mats, bowl supports and recipe book holders, as well as adapted cutlery, utensils and kitchen furniture. Elderly people with a particular disability may be able to buy aids to suit their own needs—for example, the RNIB has a range of aids for people with a visual handicap and some of these can be used in the kitchen. A local Disabled Living Centre is likely to have a display of kitchen aids and may also have the services of an occupational therapist who can give advice and assistance.

In all activities, elderly people need to be supervised, particularly in kitchen areas where there are equipment and utensils. Before using these, some elderly people may need a demonstration on the correct use so that they can work with them safely. In some instances it may be necessary to check the Health and Safety policy.

It can be an interesting project to encourage the elderly people to contribute towards a cookery book, especially if they are long-stay residents, and it can help towards fund-raising in the centre. Any activity that helps in the running of the centre should be voluntary and should complement the work already being done by the staff.

CENTRE NEWSLETTER

It may be useful to have a centre newsletter, or a group of centres may share one. This can be helpful in passing on information to the elderly people, as well as encouraging them to take a more responsible part in the running of the centre. It can be organised by a member of staff or a group of elderly people may work together to produce it. The kind of activities involved can include collecting and editing information, typing, writing articles, drawing sketches or cartoons, compiling crosswords, puzzles or competitions, having a question and answer column, finding out what is on or available in the area, noting any local items of interest, and encouraging other elderly people to contribute; lastly there is the duplicating and distributing of the newsletter. A photocopying machine can be invaluable for copying or enlarging a newsletter, though it may be possible to use carbon paper if a machine is not available. A newsletter may be produced monthly or quarterly or less often, depending upon the amount of information available and the needs of the people using the centre.

Sample of some of the items which may be included in a centre newsletter.

Centre Newsletter

Spring 1990   No. 3

Dear All,

We hope that you enjoyed the recent visits to Skegness and Derbyshire and that you are looking forward to the holiday in the summer. Thankyou for all the contributions to the Newsletter - any reader's letters not included in this issue will be mentioned in the next one, Editor.

From the staff...

The plans for the new extension to Highfields Centre have been agreed so there may be some disruption during September when one of the day rooms will need to be closed.

Harvest Festival

The Minister will be holding the Harvest Festival earlier this year - can you let staff know if you want to contribute anything towards this.

Smile awhile

At a recent nativity play in the village, one little girl was heard to exclaim that she was taking the part of Joe Smith !

Concert

A concert has been arranged at the Highfields Centre on Monday, 7th July, at 3p.m. - can you let staff know if you would like to go so that transport can be arranged.

Snooker

The Snooker Competition will be held in the Broadacres Centre during May - please let Mrs. Griffeths know if you will be entering this year.

Library Service

Good news for readers! The librarian will be visiting again during March to change the books in all the centres - please let her know if there are any particular books which you would like to read.

Crossword

Joe Crosby has compiled the new crossword (overleaf) - answers to the last crossword are also included.

What's on

There will be an 'Old Time Musical Hall' at the Alhambra Theatre on May 14th at 7.oo p.m. Facilities are now available for wheelchair users so if you would like to go, please can you let the staff know by April 10th.

Minibus

It has been agreed that all the centres are to contribute towards a minibus which can be used for outings etc.

Films

A list of forthcoming films at the local cinema has been put up on all the noticeboards.

Reader's letters ...

Dear Editor,

I would like to ask why the Domino Match was cancelled this year. I really enjoy playing the game and was very disappointed at the news.

Phyllis Johnson.

(We regret that the match had to be cancelled, Mr. Jeffries, the organiser had to leave suddenly during August and we were unable to find a replacement in time. The match for this year will be held as usual).

Roadworks

A warning to residents who may have a visual problem - the pavements on Walkley Street and Howarth Row leading to the park will be blocked during August, please can you use the opposite pavement if you are using this route.

Friends of Broadlands Centre

The Friends of Broadlands Centre would like to thank everyone who contributed to their fund-raising event in October.

CONCERTS

Concerts play an important part in the life of a centre, particularly if the elderly people are resident there. They range from formal ones given by professional musicians to quite informal productions organised by local volunteers; they may even be put on by the staff or the elderly people themselves.

A concert may include music played or sung, songs in which the audience can take part, comedy, drama, stories, poems, monologues or whatever talents are available. It may be organised around a theme such as old time music hall, or it may be held to celebrate a special occasion.

It helps to get to know local people or groups who can provide entertainment—a choir, an ensemble, a band or orchestra, bellringers, dancers, a school, college or church group, a comedian, a magician, a pianist, a singer, or perhaps a mixture of several different talents. After a while you will get to know which acts the elderly people enjoy most and can ask them to visit again.

The facilities needed for a concert vary according to the nature of the performers and the size of the audience. You will probably need a large room, a piano, chairs (with arms) for the elderly people, access for wheelchairs, extra seating for visitors and somewhere for the entertainers to use as a dressing room. The room should be well lit, heated and have sufficient ventilation. You may also need additional items such as songbooks and music.

In any activity involving groups of people it is essential to ensure that there is easy access for everyone—for the elderly people to leave the room if necessary and for staff to reach someone who needs their help. This may mean additional aisles through the audience (wide enough for wheelchairs), which are essential if everyone has to be evacuated in an emergency.

Before the concert begins, staff may like to say a few words of introduction, perhaps giving the names of the entertainers; they may also like to call for a vote of thanks afterwards.

After the concert refreshments may be provided; these are usually welcomed by the entertainers and the audience, and also give everyone a chance to meet each other. Some entertainers may charge a fee for their services while others will ask for nothing. As most entertainment does involve cost of some kind, it is worthwhile having a fund so that money is available for this purpose.

COMMITTEES

A committee representing the elderly people can be very helpful in running a centre, especially if the members are alert and able and the meetings are well organised and active. A staff member may need to be included to guide the meetings and also to organise certain aspects of an activity, such as arranging transport, sending for tickets or checking that amenities are suitable for disabled and elderly people.

The committee can be structured like any other, with a chairman, a secretary to take notes and a treasurer who will keep a record of any funds. If there are any particular groups of people attending the centre, such as those with a visual impairment or an ethnic minority, they should be asked to put forward a representative. An agenda may be drawn up or meetings may be organised informally—points to raise from people attending the centre, or information which the staff would like to pass on. Meetings may also include discussion about events to be organised and any other points of interest.

The kinds of activity in which the committee can become involved include making arrangements for outings and collecting names and payments; running activities like bingo sessions and preparing the room and equipment; asking for slide, film and video shows and suggesting speakers for talks and demonstrations; and also fund-raising activities such as helping to organise bazaars, sales of work and jumble sales and running raffles and other events. Smaller tasks may include reading a newspaper to someone who is visually impaired or writing letters, or assisting staff with other duties in the running of the centre.

Perhaps one of the most useful functions of a committee is that the members can collect information, views and criticisms from the people attending the centre and pass these on to the staff. This is especially helpful in a centre which has large numbers of people attending on different days, and only a limited number of staff.

When a committee is formed, there is likely to be a need for some form of rules, so that guidelines can be followed in electing members and setting a limit to the term of office. Meetings may be held regularly or irregularly depending on the needs of the centre, and as often as necessary. In a day centre a monthly meeting may be appropriate, while in a long-stay unit a quarterly meeting may be enough. If the centre has a different group of people attending on each day of the week, a separate committee may be needed for each day.

Some elderly people may have a particular skill which they can use in a committee, and if this can be utilised it will be rewarding for them as well as helpful to the centre. They may be good at organising other people, or be able to lead a meeting, take notes, liaise with staff, be responsible for money, or simply have a capacity to contribute in some way.

The need for an elderly people's committee will vary from centre to centre. In some it may be very successful and make a useful contribution to the running of the centre, while in others it may be difficult to organise, particularly if the elderly people are frail or confused, or unable to tackle the work involved.

EXHIBITION, SALE OF WORK OR FAIR

An exhibition or sale of work

This can be an important event in the life of the centre; it gives the elderly people an interest and a reason for collecting or making items during the year.

If work is to be exhibited, staff should try to make a special occasion of it, with prizes and perhaps a person of some standing to present them. A local photographer can be commissioned to take photographs of the exhibits or presentations, which can later be enlarged and hung in the centre.

Preparation for this kind of activity requires a lot of effort on the part of the staff, but usually it is all worthwhile, a day for the elderly people to enjoy each year.

When planning an exhibition or sale of work you should consider the following points: the size of the room or rooms where the work will be displayed; the size and number of tables and chairs and any other displays; the space required for the visitors and the elderly people (who may be in wheelchairs); and fire regulations. Posters for display in local shops and public buildings will have to be made or copied, as well as signs for the different crafts and labels for each item. If these are not being judged, the person's name can be used; otherwise they can be numbered. These labels must be fixed securely as items can easily be lost or mislaid. Award cards can be bought, and prizes will also need to be purchased. You may want to run to cups or shields which would need engraving.

Tables and other surfaces look better if covered with sheets, material or paper, and display boards can be covered with material and placed on top of the tables to hold exhibits. On some surfaces a staple gun or drawing pins can be used to attach coverings. The exhibits can be pinned onto the material on the display boards or hung or laid on the table. Try to show them off to their best advantage—badly made items can often be camouflaged. Staff may also like to trim the tables with decorations.

On the day itself activities should take place at pre-arranged times—for example, judging at 1 p.m., opening at 2 p.m. and the presentation of prizes at 3 p.m.

Additional attractions such as background music and refreshments can all help to make it an enjoyable day. If refreshments are provided, these may need to be served in a separate room or area.

A fair

This is a bigger event to organise and usually needs a group of staff to plan it well beforehand. As well as some of the activities mentioned above, there may be games and fund-raising stalls such as a white elephant stall, a second-hand book stall, a plant stall, a cake stall, a toy stall and so on. You could also have a tombola session, raffles, guessing the weight of a cake and much more. When organising a fair you may have to recruit relatives, carers and volunteers as well as staff to man the stalls, supervise the elderly people, organise the refreshments, collect and count the money, relieve others on duty and do any other tasks that may be necessary. You may also have to decide whether to hold the fair inside or outside; if you choose out-of-doors you will need to make some provision for rain.

Refreshments can be more ambitious, and you may be able to ask a local band to come and play, all adding to the atmosphere of the occasion. Bunting displayed around the centre will help to set the scene and will also advertise the event.

If the elderly people can become involved in the preparation and organising of activities, it will not only be helpful to you but will give them a sense of purpose.

FLOWER ARRANGING

This interesting and absorbing craft can offer much variety, depending upon the skill and enthusiasm of the arranger. Many books have been written about flower arranging, and these include useful instructions not only on fresh and dried flowers, but also on flowers made out of other materials such as silk, plastic and paper. Some also include information about pressed flowers for anyone who is interested in making pressed flower pictures or greetings cards.

Some elderly people may be able to attend flower arranging demonstrations organised by a local flower arranger's society, or to visit a national show. Some may even be able to attend evening classes and learn from trained teachers how to create professional and artistic arrangements. The National Association of Flower Arrangement Societies (NAFAS) is involved in organising shows and demonstrations and also issues a quarterly magazine giving useful information and listing forthcoming events. If any elderly people are unable to leave the centre, a local flower arranger may be willing to visit occasionally and give a demonstration.

Basic equipment for the craft could include a selection of different containers, pin holders to support the flowers and special 'putty' to hold them in place, 5cm fine gauge wire netting, 'oasis' which can be soaked in water (for fresh flowers), 'oasis' which does not need soaking (for dried flowers) and clippers. Those who are more ambitious and want to make an arrangement around a theme may need additional materials for their display.

Once the flowers have been bought (or picked from the garden) and the equipment obtained, the flower arranger has everything she needs to enjoy a light hobby that would be ideal for someone unable to attempt more strenuous activities. The finished arrangements will also make the centre a more attractive place and give pleasure to other elderly people using it, including those with a visual impairment who may be able to feel and smell the flowers. If an arranger has the use of only one hand, the container can be placed on a non-slip mat before the arrangement is started.

For those interested in pressing flowers, a complete flower pressing kit is available from Specialist Crafts, and the same company also makes flower presses in small, medium and large sizes. It is also possible to achieve excellent results by placing the flowers between the pages of an old telephone directory with a heavy weight on top of it.

INDOOR GARDENING

If someone enjoys gardening but is unable to go outside, indoor gardening may be the answer. This is an enjoyable pastime and can be made more interesting by having different kinds of plants and a range of containers around the centre—potted plants on a shelf or window ledge (or in a window box), in a plant stand or in a large container on the floor. It may also be possible to install a bottle garden or a terrarium (fishtank garden).

Some of the activities demand skill and you may have to split these up so that they can be done by different people. One person can choose seeds or take cuttings, another can prepare the soil or containers, another set the seeds or the cuttings and yet another can feed and care for the plants afterwards. Indoor gardening can be done by someone who has limited vision or from a wheelchair, and it is ideal for an elderly person who lacks the stamina to attempt outdoor gardening.

The equipment used need not be expensive and is usually available from the local garden centre. You will need clay or plastic plant pots (6.5cm, 9cm, 13cm and 18cm have been found to be the most useful sizes), drip saucers, fertiliser, pest killer, potting compost, secateurs, string, stakes, an old fork and spoon, a soft sponge for washing leaves, a mister for spraying plants and a watering-can. Small lightweight watering-cans are now available with a broad, stable base and those with an extended spout are particularly useful for people in wheelchairs. If someone is liable to spill the water, it may be better to use a mister or a container with a lid—an old teapot is ideal for this purpose. Visitors may be willing to bring in plant pots and other equipment that they no longer need.

Other aids include a fitted tray on a wheelchair, non-slip mats under the containers, labels with braille markings and tools with adapted handles. If a worktop is being used, it may need to be secured, and you should also check that it is at a convenient height for people who are sitting down or in a wheelchair.

Flowering plants which may be grown indoors include African violet, azalea, begonia, Busy Lizzie, flowering cacti, campanula, chrysanthemums, cyclamen, pelargonium, poinsettia and primula. Non-flowering foliage plants may also be grown. Someone who cannot see easily will appreciate scented plants such as gardenia or jasmine.

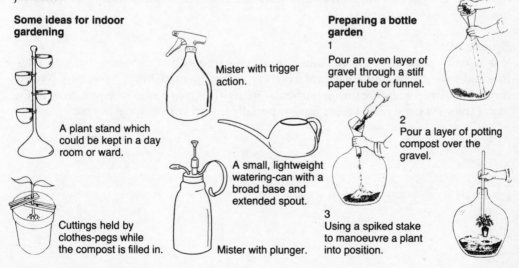

Some ideas for indoor gardening

A plant stand which could be kept in a day room or ward.

Mister with trigger action.

A small, lightweight watering-can with a broad base and extended spout.

Cuttings held by clothes-pegs while the compost is filled in.

Mister with plunger.

Preparing a bottle garden

1
Pour an even layer of gravel through a stiff paper tube or funnel.

2
Pour a layer of potting compost over the gravel.

3
Using a spiked stake to manoeuvre a plant into position.

OUTDOOR GARDENING

Outdoor gardening can be an interesting and absorbing hobby for anyone who is sufficiently able, and the flowers and produce can be used to benefit the centre. If possible the garden should be near to the centre where facilities are available, and so that staff can keep an eye on the elderly people and be on hand if any problems arise.

It is possible to plan a garden to suit the needs of elderly people, and information can be obtained on the subject so that any alterations can be made. Horticultural Therapy and the Disabled Living Foundation will both supply helpful leaflets and advice (see Appendices for addresses). Non-slip ramps can be built (a minimum incline of 1:12), paths that are wide, firm and level enough to take wheelchairs, broad, shallow steps so that a walking frame can be used on them, and handrails can be fitted by ramps and paths and in other areas where they may be needed. Raised edges on paths help to prevent wheelchairs from slipping off, and raised beds will be easier for elderly people who find bending down difficult. These can be specially designed and constructed in brick, stone, concrete or wood, or they may be tall, portable containers which can be set up in various places around the garden or on paved areas. If a garden is not available, hanging baskets or window boxes will provide interest.

If a greenhouse is to be included in the garden or on a paved area, it, too, will need to be suitable for elderly people, allowing access for wheelchairs and fitted with worktops that are firm, strong and of a convenient height. A water or electricity supply may be an advantage, and perching stools can be provided for those who are unable to stand for long periods. When siting a greenhouse, look for a sunny area, not too exposed, which has good access to supplies and is preferably near to the centre. If space is limited, a lean-to greenhouse may still be useful, particularly if easy access is required.

Some centres may have a special room or a shed which can be used to store tools, equipment and materials. This should not be too far away from the garden so that the elderly people can reach it easily.

Benches can be positioned in various places so that people can rest or view the garden. Any structures in the garden should be safe and strong, since elderly people may need to hold on to them for support.

Gardening can be enjoyed by people with several different handicaps, and also by those whose sight is failing, although it may need special adaptations for a person who has severe visual impairment.

Equipment
It is usually possible to obtain most pieces of gardening equipment, such as long-handled tools, from your local garden centre, although occasionally you may have to contact the firms manufacturing particular items. The two pieces of equipment at the top of the next page have been found especially useful with elderly people:

Perching stool

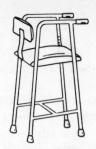

Kneeler

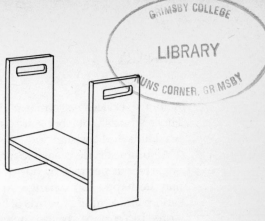

This is a high seat which may have an adjustable seat as well as a backrest and arms. The one shown is made by Ellis, Son and Paramore Ltd.

This can be used as a stool or a kneeler and can be made from wood or tubular steel. It is useful for an elderly person who can sit or kneel while working.

Long-handled tools

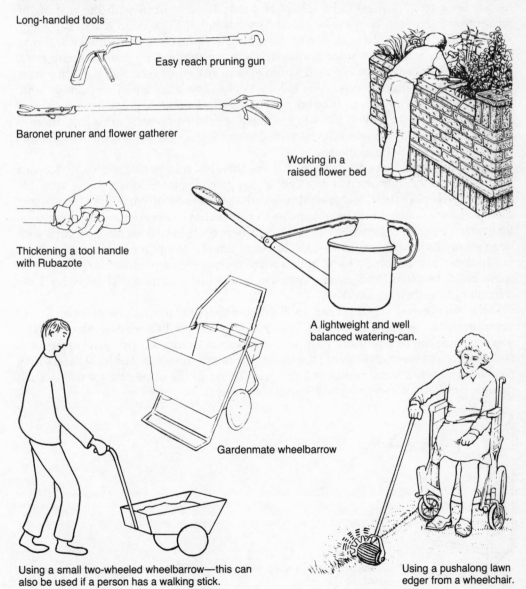

Easy reach pruning gun

Baronet pruner and flower gatherer

Working in a raised flower bed

Thickening a tool handle with Rubazote

A lightweight and well balanced watering-can.

Gardenmate wheelbarrow

Using a small two-wheeled wheelbarrow—this can also be used if a person has a walking stick.

Using a pushalong lawn edger from a wheelchair.

LIBRARY

A library service is essential in a centre where many of the elderly people enjoy reading. Those who ask for a book are usually able to manage on their own, although some will need aids and assistance.

A library service is easy to maintain once started and can normally be managed by a volunteer or perhaps by one of the elderly people themselves. The local public library may be happy to exchange books at intervals and may give advice on setting up a service and keeping records of books loaned out, returned and requested. Books can be stored in a cupboard or on shelves, and a book trolley is useful in a centre where some of the elderly people may not be mobile. It can also be used to store magazines, talking book tapes, reading aids, newspapers and any other material that needs passing round. Book trolleys need to be robust and may have to fit in with the rest of the furniture in the centre. They can be ordered from hospital, library and school suppliers.

Some elderly people have difficulty in reading the print in normal books and may manage better with large print books which are published by several companies. Magnifying aids can also be supplied to make the print easier to see. People with a more severe visual impairment may enjoy talking books. These are taped versions of well-known books and can be bought or borrowed from the local library. Most can be played on a normal cassette player, but some require special equipment for which there is usually a charge. The cassettes can be played to a group of people, or used in individual cassette players with headphones.

If any other aids are needed, an occupational therapist may be able to give advice, or a librarian or the local Disabled Living Centre may provide ideas. Bookrests are available for use in bed or in a chair, and special tables are also manufactured. Some of these have a ledge and are adjustable in height and angle; others have swivel legs which are useful for fitting around or in between chairs. Pageturners come in various forms to cope with degrees of disability; a rubber thimble on a finger, or on the end of a stick or headpointer, is the simplest form, but there are also simple pageturners for people with some hand function, and more expensive electronic models for those who have difficulty using their hands at all.

Some people enjoy being read to from newspapers, magazines or books, and volunteers can be asked to do this. Other elderly people like reading aloud, and a reading circle can be a pleasant pastime, each person having a copy of the same book and reading a passage in turn until the chapter or story is finished. The local library may be able to supply several copies of large print books of the same title for use in such groups, or the book can be passed round the group.

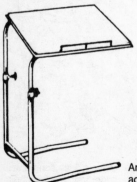

An open-ended table which slides easily under chairs. Both height and angle are adjustable.

MUSIC

Music can provide a lot of fun in a centre, particularly for confused elderly people who may be unable to take part in many of the other activities. Sing-songs, perhaps one of the most enjoyable pastimes, can entertain the most restricted person, especially if the songs are familiar to him.

Sung music is usually easier to follow if the words are written down or displayed, and if they can be blown up on a photocopier the elderly people will be able to see them more easily. The staff should know the words and tunes so that they can help everyone along. In general, the music will need to be clear, lively and louder than normal to cater for those who are partially deaf.

If there is a piano in the centre, it will add to the fun if a member of staff, a volunteer or perhaps one of the elderly people can play, particularly if some of the elderly people can dance with each other or with the staff. In centres where the people are more physically able, it may be possible to organise socials and other events.

Sometimes people will offer to visit the centre to play musical instruments, and some of the elderly people may be able to join in and either take a turn on these instruments or use instruments available in the centre, such as tambourines, triangles, drums and so on. More able people may be able to provide their own entertainment.

In some centres it may be necessary to provide some kind of entertainment throughout the day, such as television, radio, a hospital radio system or a music centre. The latter can be invaluable for a long-stay resident, enabling staff or the elderly people to put on records, tapes or the radio, whichever is preferred. Individual radio-cassettes can be bought for use in areas where people may want to be quiet while others can enjoy a tape of their choice.

A good selection of singalong videos, tapes, sheet music and song books is available in shops or by mail order, including large print song books for those with less than perfect sight.

MUSIC AND MOVEMENT

In a centre an activity like this can provide beneficial exercise for elderly people, as well as encouraging them to be sociable.

When arranging the group, you will need to look at the numbers of people involved in relation to the size of the room and the number of staff available. You must also consider their disabilities and abilities and ensure that the activity is appropriate for them and the skills of the staff leading the group. Between seven and fifteen people has been suggested as suitable for a music and movement session, although the numbers may vary depending on the independence of the elderly people and the amount of supervision and assistance they need. Before asking them to take part in the group, find out whether they have a condition that could be affected by the exercises, or whether their behaviour is likely to interfere with the running of the group.

It is usual for the elderly people to be sitting down during the session, as there is always a risk that some people may fall if they do exercises while standing. Ordinary chairs can be used, although chairs with armrests are safer. People in wheelchairs can normally join in.

The group is arranged in a circle or semi-circle, with the chairs spaced at least two armlengths apart so that no one gets injured. The leader can sit inside the circle or in front of the semi-circle to demonstrate the exercises. How much space is required will depend on the number of people taking part, and you should check the fire regulations to make sure that you are not exceeding the maximum number permitted for safety. You will need one member of staff to lead the group and a second on hand to assist the elderly people and take anyone out if necessary; she can also help in an emergency. Additional staff may be needed if the elderly people are very dependent.

The exercises should be well planned and suitable for people who are sitting down. Take care that an elderly person is not asked to do an exercise that is beyond his ability. It is a good idea to start with breathing and limbering up exercises before building up to more strenuous activity. Simple, slow exercises can be alternated with quicker ones demanding more agility, and different parts of the body can be used in consecutive exercises so that the elderly people do not tire too easily. You can include exercises involving the head, neck, shoulders, elbows, wrists, hands and fingers, and also the trunk, hips, knees, ankles, feet and toes, although hip exercises will be limited if a person is sitting down. Household and other tasks can be used to make the session more interesting and to encourage a wider range of movement—for example, pretending to wipe the door, wall, ceiling and so on. A cloth can be used to add authenticity to the movement.

You can also make use of equipment such as balls, beanbags and hoops; these can be passed from person to person, across the circle or can be part of an individual exercise. You may need special equipment for anyone who has a specific disability—for example, padded balls with bells for partially sighted people.

Any music for the group should be planned in advance so that it fits in with the exercises and the session runs smoothly. You may need to make special tapes for the different sessions by taking music from other tapes and records and recording it in sequence onto a blank tape. The rhythm and tempo of the music should be appropriate for each exercise, and you will find that music that has a definite beat and is not too fast is most suitable for elderly people. They will respond best to music that is familiar to them—indeed, if you can use old time songs you may get them to join in with the singing.

If the elderly people have not done this kind of activity before, it would be best to start with short sessions of ten to fifteen minutes each, gradually building up to longer ones, but a session of forty minutes is usually long enough.

The importance of supervision cannot be overstressed: members of the group could easily fall or feel tired or unwell. If this happens, encourage the elderly person to rest or leave the group, but a good preventive measure is to have one or two intervals during the session, so that people can relax.

Exercises that can be done from a sitting position

CLAPPING

Clap in front (several times).
Clap above head.
Clap below (clap to side).

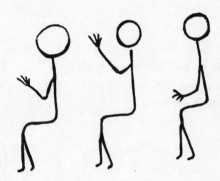

KNEES

Tap knees (several times).
Clap (several times).
Tap knees.
Clap.

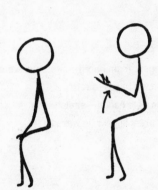

SHOULDERS

Tap left shoulder with right arm out (several times).
Left arm out (several times).
Cross over with both hands.

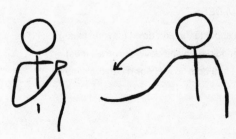

LEGS

Stretch right leg outwards.

Down (several times).

Repeat with left leg.

Alternate legs.

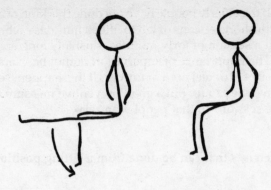

WRIST

Right wrist up and down (several times).

Left wrist up and down (several times).

Both wrists up and down.

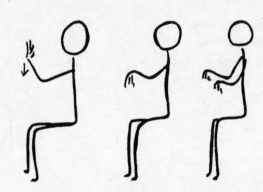

FINGERS

Grasp fingers (right hand)—stretch (several times).

Fingers in left hand—stretch.

Fingers in both hands—stretch.

Move different fingers (in waves).

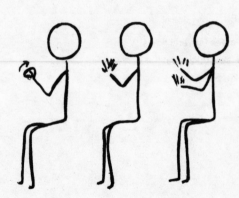

SHOULDERS

Right shoulder up and down (several times).

Left shoulder up and down (several times).

Both shoulders up and down (several times).

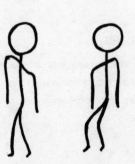

120

WRISTS

Hold right elbow in left hand.

Turn right wrist in a circle one way—other way (several times).

Turn left wrist.

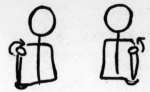
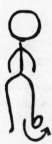

FEET

Turn right foot in a circle (several times).

Turn the other way.

Turn left foot in a circle (several times).

Turn the other way.

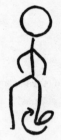
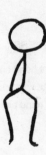

SHOULDERS

Stretch right arm sideways—down (several times).

Stretch left arm sideways—down (several times).

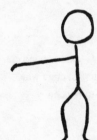

SHOULDERS

Tap fingers together—out (several times).

Stretch arms outwards with hands facing upwards—back (several times).

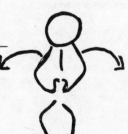
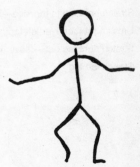

SHOULDERS

Keep hands back to back.

Stretch arms in arc outwards—back
(several times).

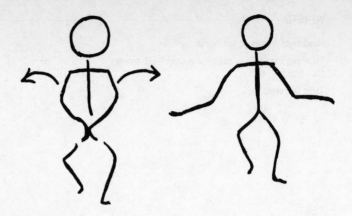

KNEES

Lift right knee upwards—down (several times).

Lift left knee up—down (several times).

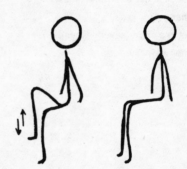

SHOULDERS

Put right hand on right shoulder—elbow facing out.

Turn elbow in a circle (several times) other way.

Put left hand on left shoulder—turn elbow.

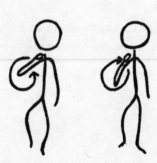

HIPS

Stretch right leg to the side—back (several times).

Cross right foot over left foot.

Stretch right leg out—(several times).

Stretch left leg.

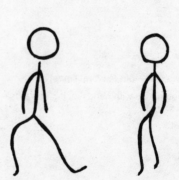

FEET

Point toe (right foot).

Right foot on heel.

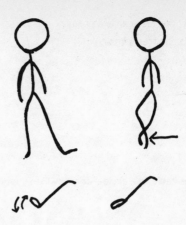

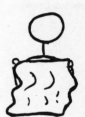

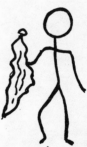

Exercises using a scarf

Hold scarf with top corners.

Shake (as if shaking a cloth).

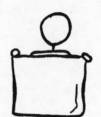

Hold one corner of scarf in right hand—let it drop.

Move scarf upwards shaking it—lower gently (several times).

Left hand.

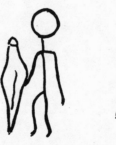

Hold the scarf with two hands up to the nose.

Move head backwards and forwards touching scarf again (several times).

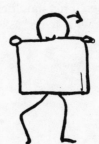

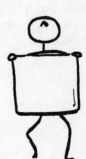

Pretend that the scarf is a duster.
Clean a shelf (as if ironing).

Clean a 'table' in a circle—one way then the other way.

Clean a 'window'. Circle one way then other way (several times)

Clean the 'ceiling'.

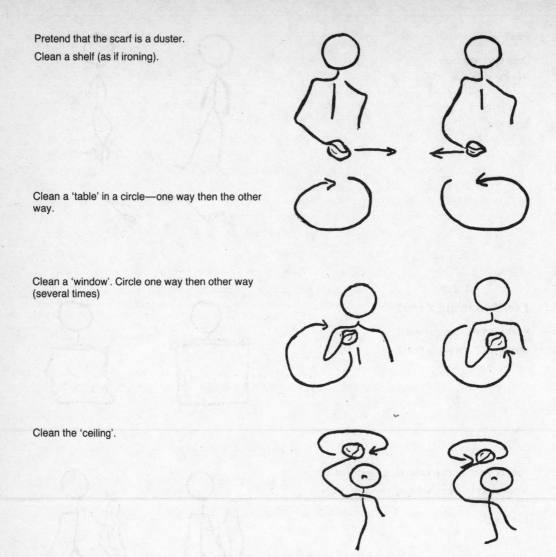

It is important that an elderly person should not be asked to try and do an activity that could aggravate his condition or cause stress or discomfort. In a music and movement group this might happen if his shoulder was stiff and painful as a result of a stroke. If you are in doubt about what to do, ask a doctor or therapist for advice before starting the session.

OUTINGS

In some centres outings may be arranged—these are particularly important in residential homes. They provide an opportunity to meet other people as well as to take part in activities outside the centre. You could organise visits to a church, a pub, shops, a community centre, the cinema, theatre or concert hall, a park or recreation area, a tea-room or a café; or to take part in a bowling match, to go fishing, attend a further education course or to visit an exhibition, craft fair or flower festival. Outings lasting several hours could be arranged to the coast or countryside, or a holiday lasting several days or longer. Sometimes exchange plans can be made, whereby elderly people from one centre can exchange for a short period with those living in another centre.

Before making any arrangements, you need to consider the following points:

—Who is well enough to go?
—Where would they like to go?
—Will the elderly people be paying their own expenses or will these come out of centre funds?
—Is transport available and is it suitable for people in wheelchairs?
—Is the driver qualified to drive the vehicle?
—Are there enough escorts?
—Are tickets required?
—Is the chosen destination suitable for elderly and disabled people—for example, could a person in a wheelchair reach and use all the facilities such as toilets and refreshment areas?
—Should anyone be notified about the visit?
—Are there adequate stopping places on the way with access to toilets for disabled people?
—Is a National Key Scheme key available? (Keys can be obtained from local Social Services Departments or from RADAR who also have lists of toilets.)
—Are any additional items needed—for example, urinal, bucket, towel, blanket, tissues, first aid materials and perhaps tablets?

Many factors may need to be considered, but it is as well to plan in advance so that everything runs smoothly on the day.

In some centres the elderly people may be able to help organise the outing by taking names of people who would like to go and any payments required.

Take care when choosing escorts if they are not staff members. They should be no younger than 18 and no older than 65, and you should ask for references if they are not relatives or friends of the elderly people. Some centres require escorts to sign a form saying that they will be responsible for the person in their care during the day. They should be fit, caring, responsible people, and remember that they may need training in the care and handling of an elderly person. You may also have to show them how to use a wheelchair and other equipment correctly. How many escorts you take on the outing will depend on the abilities of the elderly people themselves. If most of them are in wheelchairs or have mobility problems, then one escort per person is likely to be needed; if the elderly people are more able you will need fewer escorts, but you should ask the elderly people to stay in groups so that they can be supervised more easily.

When going on an outing, you must choose a suitable vehicle and check that a lift is available if it will be carrying wheelchair users. You will also need harnesses for people in wheelchairs, and clamps to fasten the wheelchairs to the floor of the vehicle.

Elderly people need adequate clothing when they go out, and this is particularly important for people in wheelchairs who may have to sit for long periods in cold and draughty areas. Special clothing is available for this purpose, made in waterproof or showerproof materials.

You can find out about access from RADAR who supply lists, and you can simplify the problem of getting the elderly people from the vehicle to the place you are visiting by using the Orange Badge parking scheme. This national scheme allows disabled drivers and passengers to park in areas normally prohibited to vehicles, such as free and unlimited parking at on-street parking meters and in time-limited waiting areas, and for two hours on single or double yellow lines if there are no double white lines in the centre of the road. Anyone using this scheme must park safely and not cause an obstruction. The scheme is available to severely disabled people who use a car owned by a government department or have a grant towards a car, receive a mobility allowance, are registered blind or have a permanent and substantial disability which causes very considerable difficulty in walking.

If an outing is planned from a day centre you will need to make arrangements for returning the elderly people to their homes at night, and remember that, whatever activity you choose, you must follow the guidelines laid down by the organisation responsible for the centre.

RECALL

Many elderly people enjoy reminiscing, and a recall group can be a good way for them to get together and have a discussion, particularly if a member of staff can lead the group.

Initially you might try a session with a fairly small group of people who are alert and can see and hear, although later on you may be able to include more people and those with disabilities.

To start the session, an old time music tape or record will help to get people in the mood and put them at ease with each other. The Education Department of Help the Aged has a selection of tapes, slides and notes which correspond with different periods from the First World War onwards. These will help to remind the elderly people about the different events in their childhood and will also help an inexperienced group leader. After showing the slides, you can put a blank tape on the tape recorder to record the discussions that follow. This will help to remind the leader of what has been said and may provide ideas for later discussion—it serves as a reminder of where the previous discussion ended. Sometimes elderly people may make comments during the showing of the slides, and the leader can take notes of these.

You can also get the talk flowing by producing objects from the past, or pictures of them, or by showing mementoes or photographs of past happenings. Sometimes reading from old newspapers will revive memories and encourage people to contribute to the discussion. It is also fun to compare prices and fashions with those of the present day.

To stimulate interest, your local library may be able to provide information about local history, and may have pictures and objects which can be shown to the group. The librarian may even be willing to organise a recall session herself. Local antique and junk shops, too, may have commonplace articles that can be used in discussions.

Equipment you could use might include a slide projector, a screen or plain wall and a tape recorder. A double tape recorder would enable you to transfer information from one tape to another.

The group leader should try to acquire a reasonable knowledge of the subject to be discussed before starting the session, as she may need to interject ideas when there is a lull in the conversation.

RELIGIOUS SERVICES

It may be possible to arrange for an occasional religious service to be held in the centre. This is appreciated by those elderly people who are unable to attend their local church or chapel. A minister or priest from one of the main Christian denominations can be asked to officiate, and if the service is kept simple it is usually acceptable to most of those who attend. If you have people from other faiths attending the centre, it may be possible to arrange services for them also.

The service can be held on a Sunday or another day of the week, and may be weekly, monthly or less frequent, depending on the availability of the minister. You may be able to organise a rota of ministers who will visit at different times.

Arrangements for a service can be quite simple—a quiet room or area, a piano, a table with a cloth, and a standing cross and flowers if these are available. If you have no piano in the centre, the minister may be able to bring a portable organ and perhaps an organist and members of his own congregation to help with the singing. You will need to provide the pianist or organist with a music edition of the hymnbooks distributed to the elderly people, and have spare hymnbooks for staff and visitors. If some of the elderly have a visual impairment, you may need to buy large print hymn books.

Often the minister will organise his own order of service, although he may ask if any of the elderly people would like to take part by singing a hymn, reading from the Bible, playing the piano or contributing in some other way.

If you serve refreshments after the service you will help to make it more of a social occasion and will enable the elderly people to meet the visitors.

Harvest festival

This is organised in the same way as any other service, except that fruit and vegetables will have to be bought or brought in by the elderly people or their visitors. These can be arranged on plates and put on the improvised altar. The minister will usually give a harvest service, and you should check that you have the appropriate music and hymns. Advertise the service in advance so that the elderly people have an opportunity to make a contribution. Any produce can be given to the elderly people afterwards or used in the kitchen.

This service is well worth organising and the elderly people enjoy making a contribution.

Carol service

This is usually a simple service to organise and need not involve a minister of the church. It is often linked to other Christmas celebrations and all you will need are carol sheets that can be easily read by elderly people. If an accompanist and music are available the service will be more enjoyable. To create an atmosphere, you could sing carols round a crib or have one or more candles in the centre of the room.

APPENDICES

APPENDICES

SOME CONDITIONS WHICH MAY BE FOUND IN ELDERLY PEOPLE

Angina

In angina, the nutrition to the heart muscle is limited. This may be due to narrowing of the blood vessels feeding the muscle, or to disease or degeneration of the heart itself. The condition is often associated with high blood pressure and rheumatic heart disease, and is found in those who overwork and lead stressful and anxious lives.

Arteriosclerosis

Hardening of the arteries, especially the middle coat of the arteries, often associated with high blood pressure. It generally affects all the arteries and can be hereditary, although it is known to be associated with anxiety, high tension of living and other stressful conditions. It usually refers to hardening of the smaller arteries.

Atherosclerosis

Degeneration which occurs mainly on the inner lining of the larger arteries, e.g. the aorta, and coronary arteries. It usually happens in later life and tends to increase with advancing age. It is sometimes associated with an excess intake of animal fats. In cerebral atherosclerosis, when the arteries of the brain are affected, there may be giddiness, loss of memory and mental changes.

Bronchitis

Inflammation of the lining of the bronchi (tubes in the lungs), which may be acute or chronic. Acute bronchitis is usually caused by bacteria and occurs most frequently in winter and foggy weather. It is especially common among the elderly. Chronic bronchitis is a condition which generally arises in people who are heavy smokers or have lived or worked in areas with severe atmospheric pollution. It manifests itself usually in the colder months, although some elderly people may have it all year round. The main symptoms are a cough, shortness of breath, especially on exertion, and wheeziness in the chest. It may be associated with heart failure. Cyanosis or blueness in the extremities may be present and there may also be oedema (collection of fluid in the tissues). Elderly people with this condition should be encouraged to keep warm and avoid smoking and getting chills.

Cataract

The lens inside the eye is transparent and the images seen are normally focused onto the retina at the back of the eye. In cataract the lens becomes partially or completely opaque and the person loses his ability to see. In the elderly this may be due to degeneration or it can be caused by injury or it may be found in a person with diabetes. An operation can be performed to improve the condition.

Diabetes

In diabetes the body's ability to regulate the amount of glucose entering the blood becomes impaired. This causes thirst, loss of energy, loss of weight and frequent passing of urine. If the condition is not treated, a person may become unconscious. Diabetes may be treated by giving a low carbohydrate diet, a diet and insulin tablets or a diet and insulin injections, depending upon the severity of the condition.

Embolism

An embolus is an obstruction in a blood vessel. It may be part of a blood clot, a bubble of air, a globule of fat or other material. It can occur in any part of the body, but is most serious when it happens in the brain (cerebral embolism), heart (coronary embolism) or in the lungs (pulmonary embolism).

Emphysema

Tends to occur in the elderly and is frequently associated with chronic bronchitis and asthma. The air sacs in the lungs become overdistended with air, and degeneration in their walls means that they have lost their elasticity. It is often connected with smoking. The symptoms are mainly those of chronic bronchitis.

Glaucoma

Occurs when there is increased pressure inside the eye. This happens when there is a build-up of fluid which is unable to drain away naturally. The condition can put pressure on the optic nerve and cause blindness.

Heart failure

Occurs when the amount of blood pumped out by the heart is too small for the needs of the body. This failure can occur in the left ventricle or chamber (left ventricular failure) or in the right ventricle (right ventricular failure).

High blood pressure

High blood pressure (hypertension) is quite a common condition, in which the blood pressure is higher than normal. The walls of the arteries may also have degenerated and thickened, and the strain on the heart to provide the body with an adequate blood supply may be greater than normal. Congestive cardiac failure may result from this condition.

Low blood pressure

Low blood pressure (hypotension) may occur naturally in some elderly people or it may be a consequence of rest or fatigue. In certain cases it may occur with a heart condition or other complaints. A person with diabetes may suffer from postural hypotension and feel faint when he tries to stand upright. In hypotension there is a limited supply of blood to the brain.

Myocardial infarction

Also known as coronary heart disease, coronary arterial disease or coronary thrombosis. The myocardium is the middle lining of the heart wall and it receives its blood supply from the coronary arteries. If the walls of these vessels become thickened and the arteries become narrow and a clot forms and blocks the flow of blood, the tissue beyond the blockage is said to be an 'infarct' or dead tissue. A person with this condition may have previously suffered from an attack of angina.

Multiple sclerosis

Multiple sclerosis (MS) or disseminated sclerosis is a chronic and progressive disease which may cause a variety of symptoms, e.g. weakness, numbness, eye conditions, etc. It affects the nerves of the brain and spinal cord where patches of scarring (sclerosis) are formed. These are usually scattered and can lead to symptoms which are unpredictable. The disease is usually discovered in younger or middle-aged people, so an elderly person with the disease is likely to have had it for some time. Remissions can occur from time to time, but are usually followed by relapses.

Osteoarthritis

Osteoarthritis (or osteoarthrosis) is a common complaint in the elderly and is caused by 'wear and tear' in the joints. It usually affects those taking the weight of the body, e.g. hips, knees or spine, and a person may complain of pain and stiffness, particularly early in the morning. He may also find that the joints 'give way' as the muscles around them become weaker through lack of use. Elderly people with this condition should be encouraged to move their joints and not remain in one position for too long.

Osteoporosis

Occurs when there is a lack of calcium in the bones. People with this condition tend to become shorter, and deformities and sometimes fractures can develop. A spinal jacket may be worn to prevent deformities in the spine. A diet rich in protein and calcium is recommended.

Paget's disease

Results in some of the bones becoming spongy and thickened and is most obvious in the skull and bowing of the legs. Deafness may occur in some cases.

Parkinson's disease

This condition was named after a doctor who first described it in 1817. It affects the part of the brain involved with movement and a person with the disease may show: fixed posture, shuffling gait, dribbling, expressionless face, difficulty in swallowing and in starting and performing movements, tremor, slurred speech and slowness of movement. The blank expression on the face can give the illusion that he is unaware of what is happening and staff need to respond to him normally and wait for his reactions. Drugs can be given to relieve the symptoms.

Pneumonia

Means inflammation of the lungs and may be 'lobar pneumonia' or 'bronchopneumonia'. In lobar pneumonia one or more lobes of a lung are affected. This tends to be an acute condition and can end in a crisis if it is not treated. It affects the air sacs in the lung, but not the bronchi or larger tubes. Bronchopneumonia affects the bronchioles or smaller tubes and can be patchy and affect both lungs. It may be secondary to another condition such as bronchitis, and occurs more often in the elderly who may be suffering from general debility and other conditions.

Rheumatoid arthritis

An inflammatory condition affecting the smaller joints, e.g. of the hands or feet, although later it may spread to the larger joints. It causes pain, swelling and stiffness in the joints and in severe cases deformities such as 'drifting' of the fingers. People with rheumatoid arthritis should try to avoid putting strain on their joints or keeping them in one position for too long. Different methods or the use of aids can make the performance of activities easier and gentle exercises can help to strengthen muscles and tendons around a joint. Splints are sometimes used to reduce deformities.

Thrombosis

Occurs when a blood clot blocks an artery or vein. It may be a coronary thrombosis (in the heart), cerebral thrombosis (in the brain) or a deep venous thrombosis (DVT) in the leg. In elderly people a DVT may happen after an operation, when bandages are applied too tightly to the leg, or may be the result of immobility.

ABBREVIATIONS

AIDS	—Acquired Immune Deficiency Syndrome	GP	—General practitioner
ATC	—Adult Training Centre	HCO	—Home care organiser
BAHOH	—British Association of the Hard of Hearing	HV	—Health visitor
		LA	—Local Authority
BASE	—British Association for Service to the Elderly	MAVIS	—Mobility Advice and Vehicle Information Service
bd	—Twice a day (medication)	MIND	—National Association for Mental Health
BDA	—British Deaf Association/ British Diabetic Association	MND	—Motor neurone disease
		MS(DS)	—Multiple sclerosis
CCF	—Congestive cardiac failure	Nok	—Next of kin
CHC	—Community Health Council	OA	—Osteoarthritis
		od	—Once a day (medication)
CN	—Community nurse	OT	—Occupational therapist
COAD	—Chronic obstructive airways disease	PHAB	—Physically Handicapped and Able-Bodied
COSHH	—Control of substances hazardous to health	POSSUM	—Patient-operated electronic selector mechanism
CPA	—Centre for Policy on Ageing	prn	—As required (medication)
		PT	—Physiotherapist
CPN	—Community psychiatric nurse	qds	—Four times a day (medication)
CRUSE	—Organisation for counselling the bereaved	RA	—Rheumatoid arthritis
CVA	—Cerebral vascular accident (stroke)	RADAR	—The Royal Association for Disability and Rehabilitation
DGH	—District general hospital	REMAP	—Rehabilitation Engineering Movement Advisory Panels
DHA	—District Health Authority		
DIAL(UK)	—Disablement Information and Advice Lines		
		RHA	—Regional Health Authority
DLF	—Disabled Living Foundation	RN	—Registered nurse
		RNIB	—Royal National Institute for the Blind
DN	—District nurse		
Dob	—Date of birth	RNID	—Royal National Institute for Deaf People
DSS	—Department of Social Security		
		SAGA	—Holidays for the elderly
DVT	—Deep venous thrombosis	ST	—Speech therapist
FHSA	—Family Health Services Authority	SW	—Social worker

| tds | —Three times a day (medication) | UTI | —Urinary tract infection |
| TIA | —Transient ischaemic attack | WRVS | —Women's Royal Voluntary Service |

BEGINNINGS AND ENDS OF WORDS

A-	—without	Hypo	—below
-able	—able to	-iasis	—condition of
-aemia	—blood	In-	—in
-aesthesia	—sensibility	Inter-	—between
-al/-an	—pertaining to	Intra-	—within
-algia	—pain	-itis	—inflammation of
Ambi-	—on both sides	-kinesia	—movement
An-	—absence of	Laryngo-	—larynx
Ante-	—before	-logy	—study of
Anti-	—opposite to	Macro-/Mega-	—large
Bi-	—two	Mal-	—abnormal
Brady-	—slow	Medi-	—middle
Broncho-	—connected with the lungs	Meta-	—between
-cardial	—heart	Micro-	—small
Cardio-	—heart	Multi-	—many
Cerebro-	—brain	My/myo-	—muscle
Co-/Con-	—together	Neo-	—new
De-	—away/from/reversing	Nephro-	—kidney
-derm	—skin	Neuro-	—nerve
-desis	—to bind together	Oculo-	—eye
Dis-	—against	-oid	—like
Dys-	—difficult/painful/abnormal	-ology	—study of
-ectomy	—removal of	-oma	—tumour
En-/End-/Endo-	—in/into/within	-opia	—eye
Ent-	—within	Ortho-	—straight/normal
Epi-	—outside	Oro-	—mouth
-esis	—action/process	Os-	—bone/mouth
Ex-	—away from	-ose	—sugar
Fore-	—in front of	-osis	—condition
Gastro-	—stomach	Osteo-	—bone
Glyco-	—sugar	-ostomy	—to form an opening
-genic	—origin of	Oto-	—ear
-graphy	—recording	-otomy	—incision of
Haema/haemo	—blood	-ous	—having nature of
Hemi-	—half	Pachy-	—thickness
Homo-	—same	Pan-	—total
Hydro-	—water	Para-	—partial/beside
Hyper-	—excess	-paresis	—weakness
		Patho-	—disease
		-pathy	—disease

Ped-	—child/foot	Semi-	—half
Per-	—by/through	Socio-	—sociology
Peri-	—around	-stomy	—to form an opening
Pharyngo-	—pharynx	Sub-	—below
-phesia	—speech	Supra-	—above
Phlebo-	—vein	Syn-	—union
-plasty	—to form	Tachy-	—fast
-plegia	—paralysis	Tarso-	—foot
Pleuro-	—covering of the lung	-therapy	—treatment
Pneumo-	—air/lung	Thoraco-	—chest
-pnoea	—breath	Thrombo-	—blood clot
Poly-	—many	Thyro-	—thyroid gland
Post-	—after	-tomy	—incision of
Pre-/pro-	—before	Tracheo-	—wind pipe
Pseudo-	—false	Trans-	—across
Psycho-	—mind	Tri-	—three
Quadri-	—four	-trophy	—nourishment
Re-	—again	Ultra-	—beyond
Retro-	—backward	Uni-	—one
Rhin-	—nose	-uria	—urine
Sclero-	—hard	Vaso-	—vessel
-sclerosis	—hardening	Veno-	—vein

USEFUL ADDRESSES

GOVERNMENT ORGANISATIONS

Department of Health, Richmond House, Room 436, 79 Whitehall, London SW1A 2NS. (Tel: 071-210 5850)

DSS Living Allowance Unit, Warbreck House, Warbreck Hill, Blackpool, FY2 0YE. (Tel: 0345 123456)

Disability Unit, Room S10/21, Department of Transport, 2 Marsham Street, London SW1P 3EB (Tel: 071-276 5255/6)

Health Education Authority, Hamilton House, Mabledon Place, London WC1H 9TX. (Tel: 071-383 3833)

Mobility Advice and Vehicle Information Services (MAVIS), Department of Transport, Crowthorne, Berkshire RG11 6AU. (Tel: 0344 770456)

Motability, Gate House, 2nd Floor, West Gate, The High, Harlow, Essex CM20 1HR. (Tel: 0279 635666)

Orange Badge Scheme, Room C10/02, Department of Transport, 2 Marsham Street, London SW1P 3EB. (Tel: 071-276 6292)

PROFESSIONAL BODIES

Central Council for Education and Training in Social Work (CCETSW). Derbyshire House, St Chads Street, London WC1. (Tel: 071-278 2455)

The Chartered Society of Physiotherapists (CSP), 14 Bedford Row, London WC1R 4ED. (Tel: 071-242 1941)

The College of Occupational Therapists, 6–8 Marshalsea Road, Southwark, London SE1 1HL. (Tel: 071-357 6480)

College of Speech and Language Therapists, 7 Bath Place, Rivington Street, London EC2A 3DR. (Tel: 071-613 3855)

The Royal College of Nursing (RCN), 20 Cavendish Square, London W1M 0AB. (Tel: 071-872 0840)

The Society of Chiropodists, 53 Welbeck Street, London W1M 7HE. (Tel: 071-486 3381)

VOLUNTARY ORGANISATIONS

Carers National Association, 20–25 Glasshouse Yard, London EC1A 4JS. (Tel: 071-490 8818)

Community Service Volunteers (CSV), 237 Pentonville Road, London N1 9NG. (Tel: 071-278 6601)

Cruse—bereavement care, Cruse House, 126 Sheen Road, Richmond, Surrey TW9 1UR. (Tel: 081-940 4818)

National Association of Volunteer Bureaux, St Peter's College, College Road, Saltley, Birmingham B8 3TE. (Tel: 021-327 0265)

National Council for Voluntary Organisations (NCVO), Regents Wharf, 8 All Saints Street, London N1 9RL. (Tel: 071-713 6161)

The Volunteer Centre, 29 Lower King's Road, Berkhamsted, Hertfordshire HP4 2AB. (Tel: 0442 873311)

Winged Fellowship Trust (Holidays), Angel House, Pentonville Road, London N1 9XD. (Tel: 071-833 2594)

Women's Royal Voluntary Service (WRVS), 234–244, Stockwell Road, London SW9 9SP. (Tel: 071-416 0146)

ORGANISATIONS CONCERNED WITH ELDERLY PEOPLE

Age Concern

There are Age Concern groups throughout the United Kingdom, involved in a range of different projects concerning elderly people—providing holidays, helping around the house and giving advice and information. A wide range of literature is published to help both elderly people and their carers.

Age Concern (England), Astral House, 1268 London Road, Norbury, London SW16 4ER. (Tel: 081-679 8000)

Age Concern (Scotland), 54a Fountainbridge, Edinburgh EH3 9PT. (Tel: 031-228 5656)

Age Concern (Northern Ireland), 3 Lower Crescent, Belfast BT7 1NR. (Tel: 0232 245729)

Age Concern (Wales), 1 Cathedral Road, Transport House, 4th Floor, Cardiff, South Glamorgan CF 9SD. (Tel: 0222 371821/371566)

Other Organisations

British Association for Service to the Elderly (BASE), 119 Hassell Street, Newcastle-under-Lyme, Staffordshire ST5 1AX. (Tel: 0782 661033)

Centre for Policy on Ageing, 25–31, Ironmonger Row, London EC1V 3QP. (Tel: 071-253 1787)

Counsel and Care for the Elderly, Twyman House, 16 Bonny Street, London NW1 9LR. (Tel: 071-485 1550)

Help the Aged, St James's Walk, Clerkenwell Green, London EC1R 0BE. (Tel: 071-253 0253)

DISABILITY

General

Centre for Accessible Environments, Nutmeg House, 60 Gainsford Street, London SE1 2NY. (Tel: 071-357 8182)

DIAL UK (Disablement Information and Advice Line), 100 Park Grange Road, Norfolk Park, Sheffield S2 3RA. (Tel: 0742 727996)

Disabled Living Foundation, 380–384 Harrow Road, London W9 2HU. (Tel: 071-289 6111)

Disability Scotland, Princes House, 5 Shandwick Place, Edinburgh EH2 4RG. (Tel: 031-229 8632)

Equipment for Disabled People, The Disability Information Trust, Mary Marlborough Lodge, Nuffield Orthopaedic Centre, Windmill Road, Headington, Oxford OX3 7LD. (Tel: 0865 227591/750103)

PHAB, 12–14 London Road, Croydon CR0 2TA. (Tel: 081-667 79443)

REMAP GB, Hazeldene, Iththam, Sevenoaks, Kent TN15 9AD. (Tel: 0732 883818)

RADAR, 12 City Forum, 250 City Road, London EC1V 8AF. (Tel: 071-250 3222)

Visiting Aid Centre, The Spastics Society, 16–18 Fitzroy Square, London W1P 5HQ. (Tel: 071-387 9571)

Disabled Living Centres

These centres give information and advice on a wide range of aids and equipment for elderly people or those with disabilities. In some centres an appointment may be necessary, so it is advisable to telephone before visiting.

The Regional Disability Service, Green Park Health Care Trust, Musgrave Park, Hospital, Stockman's Lane, Belfast BT9 7JB. (Tel: 0232 669501)

Disabled Living Centre, 260 Broad Street, Birmingham B1 2HF. (Tel: 021-643 0980)

Disabled Living Centre, 8 Queen Street, Blackpool, Lancashire FY1 1PD. (Tel: 0253 21084)

Aid and Information Centre, Wales Council for the Disabled, Llys Ifor, Crescent Road, Caerphilly, Mid Glamorgan CF8 1XL. (Tel: 0222 887325/6/7)

Disabled Living Centre, The Lodge, Rookwood Hospital, Fairwater Road, Llandaff, Cardiff CF5 2YN. (Tel: 0222 566281 ext 51/66)

The William Merritt Disabled Living Centre, St Mary's Hospital, Green Hill Road, Armley, Leeds LS12 3QE. (Tel: 0532 793140/790121)

The Leicestershire Disabled Living Centre, 76 Clarendon Park Road, Leicester LE2 3AD. (Tel: 0533 700747/8)

Merseyside Centre for Independent Living, Youens Way, off East Prescott Road, West Derby, Liverpool L14 2EP. (Tel: 051-228 9221)

Centre for Disabled Living, Macclesfield District General Hospital, Macclesfield SK10 3BL. (Tel: 0625 421000)

Disabled Living, Red Bank House, 4 St Chad's Street, Manchester M8 8QA. (Tel: 061-832 3678/9)

Department of Rehabilitation, Middlesbrough General Hospital, Ayresome Green Lane, Middlesbrough, Cleveland TS5 5AZ. (Tel: 0642 850222)

N.U.T. Council for the Disabled, at The Dene Centre, Castle Farm Road, Gosforth, Newcastle upon Tyne NE3 1PH. (Tel: 091-2840480)

The Disability Centre for Independent Living, c/o Community Service Centre, Queen Street, Paisley, Strathclyde PA1 2PU. (Tel: 041-887 0597)

The Frank Sorrell Centre, Prince Albert Road, Eastney, Portsmouth PO4 9ER. (Tel: 0705 737174)

Independent Living Centre, 108 The Moor, Sheffield SW1 4DP. (Tel: 0742 737025)

Southampton Aids and Equipment Centre, Southampton General Hospital, Tremona Road, Southampton SO9 4XY. (Tel: 0703 777222 ext 3414)

Stockport Disabled Living Centre, St Thomas Hospital, Shaw Heath, Stockport SK3 8BL. (Tel: 061-419 4476)

Swindon Centre for Disabled Living, Marshgate, Stratton Road, Swindon SN1 2PN. (Tel: 0793 643966)

Specific Disabling Conditions

Action for Dysphasic Adults (ADA), 1 Royal Street, London SE1 7LL. (Tel: 071-261 9572)

Alzheimer's Disease Society, Gordon House, Greencoat Place, London SW1P 1PH. (Tel: 071-306 0606)

Arthritis Care, 18 Stephenson Way, London NW1 2HD. (Tel: 071-916 1500)

Arthritis and Rheumatism Research Council, PO Box 177, Chesterfield S41 7TQ. (Tel: 0246 558033)

British Association for the Hard of Hearing, 7–11 Armstrong Road, London W3 7JL. (Tel: 081-743 1110)

British Deaf Association, 38 Victoria Place, Carlisle CA1 1HU. (Tel: 0228 48844)

British Diabetic Association, 10 Queen Anne Street, London W1M 0BD. (Tel: 071-323 1531)

British Epilepsy Association, Anstey House, 40 Hanover Square, Leeds LS3 1BE. (Tel: 0532 439393)

British Limbless Ex-Servicemen's Association (BLESMA), Frankland Moore House, 185–187 High Road, Chadwell Heath, Romford, Essex RM6 6NA. (Tel: 081-590 1124/5)

MIND, 20–22 Harley Street, London W1N 2ED. (Tel: 071-637 0741)

Multiple Sclerosis Society, 25 Effie Road, Fulham, London SW6 1EE. (Tel: 071-736 6267)

National Association for Limbless Disabled (NALD), 31 The Mall, London W5 2PX. (Tel: 081-579 1758)

National Deaf-Blind League, 18 Rainbow Court, Paston Ridings, Peterborough, PE4 6UP. (Tel: 0733 73511)

Parkinson's Disease Society, 22 Upper Woburn Place, London WC1H 0RA. (Tel: 071-383 3513)

Partially Sighted Society, 62 Salusbury Road, London NW6 6NP. (Tel: 071-372 1551)

Royal National Institute for the Blind (RNIB), 224 Great Portland Street, London W1N 6AA. (Tel: 071-388 1266)

Royal National Institute for Deaf People (RNID), 105 Gower Street, London WC1E 6AH. (Tel: 071-387 8033)

The Stroke Association, CHSA House, Whitecross Street, London EC1Y 8JJ. (Tel: 071-490 7999)

SPECIALIST ORGANISATIONS

Many of the societies previously listed, such as the Disabled Living Foundation, provide advice, publications and equipment to help in daily living and specific activities. The societies listed below are each devoted to one particular subject.

British Chess Federation, 9a Grand Parade, St Leonards-on-Sea, East Sussex TN38 0DD. (Tel: 0424 442500)

Council for Music in Hospitals, 340 Lower Road, Little Bookham, Surrey. (Tel: 0923 252809)

Horticultural Therapy, Goulds Ground, Vallis Way, Frome, Somerset BA11 3DW. (Tel: 0373 64782)

Mobility Information Service and Disabled Motorists' Federation, Unit 2a, Atcham Estate, Shrewsbury SY4 4UG. (Tel: 0743 761889)

National Association of Flower Arrangement Societies of Great Britain, 21a Denbigh Street, London SW1V 2HF. (Tel: 071-828 5145)

SUPPLIERS OF MATERIALS AND EQUIPMENT

Wheelchairs

Bencraft Ltd, The Avenue, Rubery, Rednal, Birmingham B45 9AP. (Tel: 021-457 9001)

Huntleigh Nesbit Evans, Mobility Division, 15 Cronin Courtyard, Weldon, South Industrial Estate, Corby, Northamptonshire NN18 8AG. (Tel: 0536 267660)

Possum Controls Ltd, 8 Farnborough Close, Aylesbury Vale Industrial Park, Duck Lake, Aylesbury HP20 1DQ. (Tel: 0753 579236)

Newton Products, Meadway Works, Garretts Green Lane, Birmingham B33 0SQ. (Tel: 021-785 0355)

Raymar, Unit 1, Fairview Estate, Reading Road, Henley-on-Thames, Oxon RG9 1HE. (Tel: 0491 578446)

Remploy Wheelchairs, 11 Nunnery Drive, Sheffield S2 1TA. (Tel: 0742 757631)

Sunrise Medical Ltd, Fens Pool Avenue, Wallows Industrial Estate, Brierley Hill, West Midlands DY5 1BR. (Tel: 0384 480480)

Vessa Ltd, Paper Mill Lane, Alton, Hampshire GU34 2PY. (Tel: 0420 83294)

Aids and Clothing

Aremco, Grove House, Lenham, Kent ME17 2PX. (Tel: 0622 858502)
Cups, trays, holdalls, etc. which can be attached to wheelchairs. Leisure aids.

Comfy Products, 29 Havelock Crescent, Bridlington, East Yorkshire YO16 4JH. (Tel: 0262 676417)
Clothing.

Crelling Harnesses for the Disabled, 11–12 The Crescent East, Cleveleys, Lancs. FY5 3LT. (Tel: 0253 852298/821780)
Harnesses.

Dri Rider Ltd, The Yews, The Causeway, Mark Highbridge, Somerset TA9 4QF (Tel: 0278 64381)
Waterproof clothing.

Medipost Ltd, Patient Lifting Equipment, 100 Shaw Road, Oldham, Lancashire OL1 4AY. (Tel: 061-678 0233)
Clothing, leisure aids.

Simplantex Eastbourne Ltd, 67a Willowfield Road, Eastbourne, East Sussex BN22 8AR. (Tel: 0323 410470)
Clothing.

Three Jay & Co, 8, Nazeing Glassworks Estate, Nazeing New Road, Broxbourne, Hertfordshire EN10 6SF. (Tel: 0992 442974/463947)
Clothing.

Leisure Activities

Many of the organisations listed under 'Disability' can supply special equipment for those who have difficulty in holding objects or whose sight is impaired. The following organisations also have a large range covering many arts, crafts and games:

Anything Left-Handed Ltd, 57 Brewer Street, London W1R 3FB. (Tel: 071-437 3910)
Specialist suppliers for those who are left-handed or have no use of their right hand.

Homecraft Supplies Ltd, Low Moor Estate, Kirkby-in-Ashfield, Nottinghamshire NG17 7JZ. (Tel: 0623 754047)

Nottingham Rehab, Ludlow Hill Road, West Bridgford, Nottingham NG2 6HD. (Tel: 0602 452345)

Smit & Co. Ltd, Unit 1, Eastern Road, Aldershot, Hampshire GU12 4TE. (Tel: 0252 362626)

Arts and Crafts

C. P. Carter & Parker Ltd, Netherfield Road, Guiseley, Yorkshire LS20 9PD.
(Tel: 0943 872264)
Easy-to-read knitting patterns.

Daler Rowney Ltd, PO Box 10, Bracknell, Berkshire RG12 8ST. (Tel: 0344 424621)
Artists' materials, 'teach yourself' painting kits.

DMC Creative World Ltd, Pullman Road, Wigston, Leicester LE18 2DY.
(Tel: 0533 811040)
Embroidery materials and kits, sewing materials, magnifiers.

Readicut Wool Co. Ltd, Terry Mills, Ossett, Yorkshire WF5 9SA. (Tel: 0924 810881)
Materials for knitting, embroidery and rug-making. Knitting aids.

Specialist Crafts Ltd, PO Box 347, Leicester LE1 9QS. (Tel: 0533 510405)
Artists' materials, crafts materials.

Winsor & Newton, Whitefriars Avenue, Wealdstone, Harrow, Middlesex HA3 5RH.
(Tel: 081-427 4343)
Artists' materials.

Games

Artcoe, Anvil House, 172 Psalter Lane, Sheffield S11 8UR. (Tel: 0742 684701/2)
Blackboard paint.

Cartwright Brice & Co Ltd, Ossory Road, London SE1 5AN. (Tel: 071-237 3515)
Blackboards, flip-charts, drywipe boards.

Falcon Games Ltd, Travellers Lane, Welham Green, Hatfield, Hertfordshire
AL9 7JD. (Tel: 0707 260436)
Table games, jigsaws.

Nobo Visual Aids Ltd, Alder Close, Compton Industrial Estate, Eastbourne, East
Sussex BN23 6QB. (Tel: 0323 641521)
Blackboards, flip-charts, drywipe boards.

J. W. Spear & Sons Ltd, Richard House, Enstone Road, Enfield, Middlesex EN3 7TE.
(Tel: 081-805 4848)
Bingo, card games, table games.

Thurston, 110 High Street, Edgware, Middlesex HA8 7HF. (Tel: 081-952 2002)
Billiard and snooker tables. Advice about aids.

Gardening

The following firms supply tools which could be used by elderly people or those
with disabilities. These can also be obtained from organisations catering specifically
for people with disabilities.

Bulldog Tools Ltd, Clarington Forge, Darlington Street East, Wigan WN1 3DD.
(Tel: 0942 44281)

Gardena (UK) Ltd, Dunhams Lane, Letchworth, Hertfordshire SG6 1BD.
(Tel: 0462 686688)

Spear & Jackson Ltd, St. Paul's Road, Wednesbury, West Midlands WS10 9RA.

Stanley Tools Ltd, Woodside, Sheffield S3 9PD. (Tel: 0742 768888)

Wilkinson Sword Ltd, Fiskars (UK) Ltd, Bridgend Business Centre, Bridgend, Mid
Glamorgan CF31 3XJ. (Tel: 06566 55595)

Wolf Tools Ltd, Alton Road, Ross-on-Wye, Herefordshire HR9 5NE.
(Tel: 0989 767600)

Reading

Several firms specialise in publishing large print books. The following are a few of them. Some include large-print song books in their lists.

Chivers Press Publishers, Windsor Bridge Road, Bath, Avon BA2 3AX.
  (Tel: 0225 335336)
ISIS Large Print, 55 St Thomas Street, Oxford OX1 1JG. (Tel: 0865 250333)
Magna Large Print Books, Magna House, Long Preston, nr. Skipton, N. Yorkshire
  BD23 4ND. (Tel: 07294 225)
The Reader's Digest Fund for the Blind, Inc., Large Type Publications, P.O. Box 402,
  Mount Morris, Illinois 61054-0402, USA.
F. A. Thorpe (Publishing) Ltd, The Green, Bradgate Road, Anstey, Leicester
  LE7 7FU. (Tel: 0533 364325)

The following firm specialises in low vision aids, including a range of magnifiers:
Edward Marcus Ltd, 14 Goswell Road, London EC1M 7AA. (Tel: 071-490 5915)

A wooden book trolley is available from:
James Galt & Co. Ltd, Brookfield Road, Cheadle, Cheshire SK8 2PN.
  (Tel: 061-428 8511)

Music

Large print song books are available from some of the publishers listed above, and from Winslow Press (see 'Specialist Publishers' below). Sheet music for those with the use of only one hand is available from:
The National Music and Disability Information Service, Foxhole, Dartington, Totnes,
  Devon TQ9 6EB. (Tel: 0803 866701)

Winslow Press also produce videos and tapes for group singing (see end of Book List). Large print hymn books, and carol books are published by the same publisher, by the Partially Sighted Society (see 'Specific Disabling Conditions') and by:
HarperCollins Publishers, 77–85 Fulham Palace Road, London W6 8JB.
  (Tel: 081-741 7070)

Specialist Publishers

RIBA Publications Ltd, 39 Moreland Street, London EC1V 8BB. (Tel: 071-251 0791)
  Book on designing buildings to allow access for people with disabilities.
Scriptographic Publications Ltd, Channing House, Butts Road, Alton, Hampshire
  GU34 1ND. (Tel: 0420 541738)
  A series of easy-to-follow booklets on subjects related to disabled people and their carers.
  Minimum order 50 copies.
Winslow Press, Telford Road, Bicester, Oxon. (Tel: 0869 244733)
  A large range of books for those caring for elderly and disabled people and for the people
  themselves. Videos, cassettes, pictures and postcards and slides.

FURTHER READING

GENERAL

Directory for Disabled People, A. Darnbrough and D. Kinrade. 6th edition, Woodhead
  Faulkner, 1991.
Directory for Older People, A. Darnbrough and D. Kinrade. 2nd edition, Woodhead
  Faulkner, 1992.
Directory of Services for Elderly People. Centre for Policy on Ageing.
First Aid Manual. St John Ambulance/St Andrews Ambulance/British Red Cross.

DAY AND RESIDENTIAL CARE CENTRES

Caring for Elderly People, S. Hooker, 3rd edition, Routledge & Kegan Paul, 1990.
Centre Active: An activities guide for day centres and clubs for older people. Age Concern
  Scotland, 1988.
Centre Forward, a step-by-step guide to starting a day centre for older people. Age
  Concern Scotland, 1984.
Day Care for Older People in Day Centres, a discussion paper. Age Concern Scotland.
Designing for the Disabled, S. Goldsmith, RIBA Publications, 1984.
Giving Good Care: An introductory guide for care assistants. Help the Aged.
Good Care Management: A guide to setting up and managing a residential home, Jenyth
  Worsley, Age Concern, 1992.
Groupwork with the Elderly: Principles and practice, Mike Bender, Andrew Norris and
  Paulette Bauckham. Winslow Press, 1987.
Home Life: A code of practice for residential care. Centre for Policy on Ageing.
Making Residential Care Feel Like Home, J. Garland, Winslow Press, 1991.
Small and Beautiful, small day centres in Scotland. Age Concern Scotland.
Taking Good Care: A handbook for care assistants, Jenyth Worsley. Age Concern, 1989.
A Tale of Two Centres, the story of setting up two very different day centres. Age
  Concern Scotland.
Tell Them About It, Anne Connor. A guide to monitoring and evaluation. Age
  Concern Scotland, 1991.
Who's Caring Today? a report of a study of day care centres in Dumfries and
  Galloway. Age Concern Scotland.

FURNITURE AND EQUIPMENT

Chairs and Chair Accessories. DLF Hamilton Index.
Choosing a Chair. DLF information booklet.
Furniture. Equipment for Disabled People, The Disability Information Trust, 1992.
How to Get Equipment for Disability, Michael Mandelstam. Kogan Page and Jessica
  Kingsley for the Disabled Living Foundation, 1993.

VOLUNTARY WORKERS

The Gentle Art of Listening: Counselling skills for volunteers, Janet K. Ford and Philippa Merriman. The Volunteer Centre.
Training: One to One Support for Volunteers—some training ideas, Lisa Conway. The Volunteer Centre, 1994.
Working with Older Volunteers: A practical guide, Alan Dingle. Age Concern, 1993.

ELDERLY PEOPLE AND THEIR HEALTH PROBLEMS

General
Ageing—the Facts, N. Coni, W. Davison and S. Webster. 2nd revised edition, Oxford University Press, 1992.
Common Symptoms of Disease in the Elderly, H. M. Hodkinson, Blackwell Scientific Publications.
The Older Patient, R. E. Irvine, M. K. Bagnall and B. J. Smith, 4th revised edition, Hodder & Stoughton, 1986.
Staying Active: A positive approach in residential homes. Centre for Policy on Ageing.

Stroke
Stroke—A handbook for the patient's family, G. Mulley. The Stroke Association.
Stroke: A self-help manual for stroke sufferers and relatives, R. M. Youngson. David & Charles, 1990.

Dementia
Alzheimer's Disease, Robert T. Woods. Souvenir Press, 1989.
The Caring Manual: A guide for families and other carers. Alzheimer's Disease Society.
Dementia Care: A handbook for residential and day care, Alan Chapman, Alan Jacques and Mary Marshall. Age Concern, 1994.
Managing Common Problems with the Elderly Confused, D. Stokes. Screaming and Shouting, 1986; Wandering, 1986; Aggression, 1987; Incontinence and Inappropriate Urinating, 1987. Winslow Press.
Reality Orientation: Principles and Practice, Lorna Rimmer. Winslow Press, 1982.
Severe Dementia: The provision of long-stay care. Centre for Policy on Ageing.
Whatever Happened to Grandad?, B. Lodge. MIND.
Working with Dementia, G. Stokes and F. Goudie. Winslow Press, 1990.

Incontinence
In Control: Help with incontinence, Penny Mares. Age Concern, 1990.
Managing Incontinence, Cheryle B. Gartley. Souvenir Press, 1989.
Notes on Incontinence. DLF Hamilton Index.
Understanding Incontinence: A guide to the nature and management of a very common complaint, D. Mandelstam. Chapman & Hall for the DLF, 1988.

Visual Impairment
The In Touch Handbook: Services for people with a visual handicap. BBC Publications, 1993.

LIFTING AND MOVING ELDERLY PEOPLE

Choosing a Hoist. DLF information booklet.
Handling the Handicapped: A guide to the lifting and movement of disabled people.
   Chartered Society of Physiotherapists, 1975.
The Handling of Patients. Back Pain Association/Royal College of Nursing, 1993.
Hoists, Lifts and Lifting Equipment. DLF Hamilton Index.
Hoists and Lifts. Equipment for Disabled People. The Disability Information Trust.
Hoists and Their Use, Christine Tarling. Heinemann Medical Books.
Moving and Lifting for Carers, M. Hutchinson and R. Rodgers. Woodhead Faulkner,
   1991.

WHEELCHAIRS

Choosing an Electric Wheelchair. DLF Information booklet.
Getting the Best from Your Wheelchair. RADAR, 1992.
How to Push a Wheelchair. 8th edition, Disabled Motorists' Club, 1989.
Manual Wheelchairs. DLF Hamilton Index.
People with Disabilities. Booklet. Scriptographic Publications.
Powered Wheelchairs, Scooters and Buggies. DLF Hamilton Index.
Wheelchair Users. Booklet. Scriptographic Publications.
Wheelchairs. Equipment for Disabled People, 7th edition. The Disability Information
   Trust, 1993.

TRANSPORT

Door to Door: A guide to public transport facilities. 4th edition, HMSO, 1992.
Ins and Outs of Car Choice for Elderly and Disabled. Department of Transport, 1988.

ACTIVITIES

General
Leisure Activities. DLF Hamilton Index.

Arts and Crafts
The Complete Book of Pressed Flowers, Penny Black, Dorling Kindersley, 1988.
'Learn to Paint' series. Books on drawing, watercolours, oils and how to paint
   different subjects. HarperCollins.
Left-hander's Guide to Crochet. Booklet. Anything Left-handed Ltd.
Left-hander's Guide to Knitting. Booklet, Anything Left-handed Ltd.
Make it with Lollipop Sticks. Booklet. Nottingham Rehab.
Make it with Matchsticks. Booklet. Nottingham Rehab.
Patchwork. Avril Colby, Batsford, 1987.
The Reader's Digest Step-by-Step Guide to Sewing and Knitting. Reader's Digest, 1993.

Games
Billiards and Games. Know the Game booklet. A & C Black, 1993.
Card Games. Know the Game booklet. A & C Black.
Chess for Absolute Beginners. Ray Keene. Batsford, 1993.
Equipment and Games Catalogue. RNIB, 1993–4.

Family and Party Games. Collins Gem Guide, 1990.
Hoyle's Modern Encyclopedia of Card Games, W. B. Gibson, Robert Hale, 1993.
The New Book of Patience Games, Ruth D. Botterill. W. Foulsham & Co, 1982.
Patience Games. Know the Game. A & C Black, 1976.
The Penguin Book of Card Games, David Parlett. Penguin Books, 1993.
Pub Games. Booklet. A & C Black.

Other Activities

Household Equipment. DLF Hamilton Index.
Gardening in Retirement, Isobel Pays. Age Concern, 1985.
Gardening is for Everyone, A. Cloet and C. Underhill, Souvenir Press, 1982.
Gardening Without Sight, Kathleen Fleet. RNIB, 1989.
Wisley Handbooks. A large range of paperbacks on all aspects of gardening and plants. Cassell.
Daily Telegraph Cryptic Crosswords. Collections published every six months. Pan Books.
Daily Telegraph Quick Crosswords. Collections published every six months. Pan Books.
Jumbo Print Crossword Book, Terry Pitts-Fenby. Age Concern/Grub Street.
The Magic of Movement, Laura Mitchell. Age Concern, 1988.
Large print Song Book and Hymn Book. Ulverscroft Large Print Books.
Mission Praise Combined. Large print hymn book. HarperCollins.
Popular Carols. The Partially Sighted Society.
Song Book. 100 popular songs, hymns and carols. Winslow Press, 1994.
30 Years of Popular Music. Winslow Press, 1994.
Gardens of England and Wales Open to the Public. Annual publication. National Gardens Scheme.
Holidays in the British Isles: Guide for Disabled People. RADAR. Published annually.
Access to Public Conveniences. Separate publications for England, Scotland and Wales. RADAR.
Reminiscence and Recall: A guide to good practice, Faith Gibson, Age Concern, 1994.
Reminiscence with Elderly People, Andrew Norris. Winslow Press, 1994.
The Reminiscence Quiz Book, M. Sherman. Winslow Press, 1991.

LEAFLETS

Many of the organisations listed under 'Disability' in the Useful Addresses provide information leaflets on a wide variety of subjects. They will provide lists if required.

VIDEOS AND TAPES

'Music Memories and Milestones'. A selection of videos with music and events from the 1930s, '40s, '50s and '60s. Winslow Press, 1994.
'Dance-time'. A tape for elderly people who may be able to attempt dancing. Winslow Press, 1994.
'Music of Yesteryear'. A selection of tapes with songs from the 1920s, '30s and '40s. Winslow Press, 1994.
'Musical Quiz'. Two tapes with 80 songs which can be used for a musical quiz. Winslow Press, 1994.
'Sing Along Tape'. A tape for community singing. Winslow Press, 1994.